T0224984

SpringerBriefs in Computer Science

Series Editors

Stan Zdonik, Brown University, Providence, RI, USA

Shashi Shekhar, University of Minnesota, Minneapolis, MN, USA

Xindong Wu, University of Vermont, Burlington, VT, USA

Lakhmi C. Jain, University of South Australia, Adelaide, SA, Australia

David Padua, University of Illinois Urbana-Champaign, Urbana, IL, USA

Xuemin Sherman Shen, University of Waterloo, Waterloo, ON, Canada

Borko Furht, Florida Atlantic University, Boca Raton, FL, USA

V. S. Subrahmanian, University of Maryland, College Park, MD, USA

Martial Hebert, Carnegie Mellon University, Pittsburgh, PA, USA

Katsushi Ikeuchi, University of Tokyo, Tokyo, Japan

Bruno Siciliano, Università di Napoli Federico II, Napoli, Italy

Sushil Jajodia, George Mason University, Fairfax, VA, USA

Newton Lee, Institute for Education, Research and Scholarships, Los Angeles, CA, USA

SpringerBriefs present concise summaries of cutting-edge research and practical applications across a wide spectrum of fields. Featuring compact volumes of 50 to 125 pages, the series covers a range of content from professional to academic.

Typical topics might include:

- A timely report of state-of-the art analytical techniques
- A bridge between new research results, as published in journal articles, and a contextual literature review
- A snapshot of a hot or emerging topic
- An in-depth case study or clinical example
- A presentation of core concepts that students must understand in order to make independent contributions

Briefs allow authors to present their ideas and readers to absorb them with minimal time investment. Briefs will be published as part of Springer's eBook collection, with millions of users worldwide. In addition, Briefs will be available for individual print and electronic purchase. Briefs are characterized by fast, global electronic dissemination, standard publishing contracts, easy-to-use manuscript preparation and formatting guidelines, and expedited production schedules. We aim for publication 8–12 weeks after acceptance. Both solicited and unsolicited manuscripts are considered for publication in this series.

**Indexing: This series is indexed in Scopus, Ei-Compendex, and zbMATH **

Teik Toe Teoh

Convolutional Neural Networks for Medical Applications

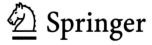 Springer

Teik Toe Teoh
Division of Information Technology &
Operations Management
Nanyang Technological University
Singapore, Singapore

ISSN 2191-5768 ISSN 2191-5776 (electronic)
SpringerBriefs in Computer Science
ISBN 978-981-19-8813-4 ISBN 978-981-19-8814-1 (eBook)
https://doi.org/10.1007/978-981-19-8814-1

This Springer imprint is published by the registered company Springer Nature Singapore Pte Ltd.
The registered company address is: 152 Beach Road, #21-01/04 Gateway East, Singapore 189721,
Singapore

Preface

This book is a compilation of research in using Convolutional Neural Networks (CNNs) for Medical Applications, written by Dr Teoh Teik Toe. It contains many publications and lessons learnt in applying CNNs during Dr Teoh's career as a Deep Learning researcher.

Dr. Teoh has been pursuing research in Big Data, Deep Learning, Cyber-security, Artificial Intelligence, Machine Learning and Software Development for more than 25 years. His works have been published in more than 50 journals, conference proceedings, books and book chapters. His qualifications include a PhD in Computer Engineering from the NTU, Doctor of Business Administration from the University of Newcastle, Master of Law from the NUS, LLB and LLM from the UoL, CFA, ACCA and CIMA. He has more than 15 years' experience in Data Mining, Quantitative Analysis, Data Statistics, Finance, Accounting and Law and is passionate about the synergy between business and technology. He believes that deep learning has a wide variety of applications and is eager to share his knowledge in applying such technologies in a wide variety of fields.

The field of Artificial Intelligence is very broad. It focuses on creating systems, capable of executing tasks which would require some form of human intelligence. In-depth knowledge and understanding of the field is required to be able to develop good Artificial Intelligence programs. Convolutional Neural Networks are a class of Artificial Intelligence algorithms which are commonly used for image data.

Throughout his career, Dr. Teoh has researched in applying deep learning to solve a variety of problems in various fields. He has extensive experience in applying deep learning in stock price prediction, medical imaging, cyber security, emotion recognition and many more.

Singapore, Singapore   Teik Toe Teoh

Acknowledgements

This book would not be possible without the hard work of the researchers that I have worked with in applying Computer Vision to Medical Imagery. I would like to give thanks to all those that have contributed to the book chapters below:

Du Yifei and Chen Zipei for putting in the hard work for the Brain Tumor and Skin Cancer Classification challenges.

Liu Jiahang, Zhao Wenkang, Li Zongyi, Song Zeyang for working diligently on the task to detect Pneumonia in afflicted children.

Shuhan Xiao, Zihan Ran, Anjie Yang for looking into classifying different White Blood Cells for the challenge.

Wenjie Guo, Mengfan Dong, Ruishu Guo, Xinnong Du, Xiuyuan Li, Yuchen Zhao for collaborating to classify diabetic retinopathy in affected patients.

I would like to thank the Springer team for the support provided from turning this book idea into reality.

Last but not least, I would like to acknowledge and thank the family and friends who have supported us throughout this journey, including all those who have helped made publishing this book possible.

Contents

Chapter 1
Introduction

As a branch of machine learning, deep learning has developed rapidly in the past two decades. The reason is that a series of neural networks with large parameters and complex structures have been established, which can be used to widely extract the characteristics of input information, thereby dividing the decision boundary more accurately. In the neural network, the convolutional neural network (CNN) is a classical and efficient network hierarchy. CNN was first proposed by Yann Lecun and applied to handwritten number recognition [7]. Its essence is a multi-layer perceptron. The reason for its success lies in the way of local connection and weight sharing, enabling effective feature extraction on images at different scales.

1.1 Medical Imaging

Medical imaging, sometimes referred to as radiography, is the area of practice where physicians make new pictures of various body areas for diagnostic or therapeutic purposes [2]. Trained experts may identify diseases and injuries without invasive procedures thanks to non-invasive testing used in medical imaging.

The development of medical imaging is among the most significant in contemporary medicine. Medical imaging procedures come in a variety of forms, including:

- X-rays
- Magnetic resonance imaging (MRI)
- Ultrasounds
- Endoscopy
- Tactile imaging
- Computerized tomography (CT scan)

Other beneficial medical imaging methods include nuclear medicine functional imaging, such as positron emission tomography (PET) scans. Scanners are an

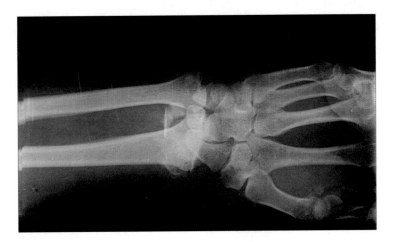

Fig. 1.1 Example of an X-ray image

example of a medical imaging application. Doctors can use scans to assess how well your body is responding to therapy for an illness or injury (Fig. 1.1).

1.1.1 Example of An X-ray Image

Medical imaging technologies are frequently used in radiography. Although X-rays and CT scans are tremendously helpful, they must be utilized cautiously owing to the ionizing radiation they emit. Ionizing radiation exposure increases the risk of cancer, cataracts, cellular mutation, and improper fetal development. However, since MRIs don't use ionizing radiation, they provide lower hazards. One of the safest modalities of medical imaging is ultrasound, which produces pictures using ultrasonic vibrations.

Surface-mounted sensors, which monitor electrical activity, are another safe type of medical imaging. Even though they provide a graph showing changes over time rather than a picture, they are often employed in electroencephalography (also known as EEG) and electrocardiography (also known as ECG).

Artificial intelligence (AI) is now being utilized in a variety of medical imaging technologies to assist in the interpretation and analysis of test data. In the area of AI known as computer vision, methods are used to visually diagnose diseases that a human eye might miss.

1.1.2 Users of Medical Imaging

A medical imaging technologist or otherwise known as a radiographer, are in charge of conducting medical imaging procedures. Radiographers are trained in universities with an in-depth understanding about the structure of the body and how it is affected by various diseases and injuries. They can specialize in medical imaging procedures, such as MRIs and CT scans, as well as other areas such as:

- Angiography which involves imaging the blood vessels and heart of a patient.
- Mobile radiography which uses specialised machines to perform imaging procedures on patients that are too ill to visit a hospital.
- Fluoroscopy which uses x-ray to analyze the patient's internal body and visualizes moving images on a screen, similar to a movie.
- Trauma radiography which frequently involves work in emergency departments.

Radiographers perform medical imaging procedures once requested by a radiologist. Radiologists are medical professionals trained to diagnose and cure diseases and injuries through the use of medical imaging. They are also in charge of treating diseases such as cancer and heart disease, using radiation or minimally invasive image-led surgery.

Once the imaging process is complete, the radiographer presents the developed images to the radiologist. The radiologist would evaluate the results, present a diagnosis of the disease or injury and determine the best treatment options for the patient.

1.1.3 Importance of Medical Imaging

Doctors can better assess patients' bones, organs, tissue and blood vessels using non-invasive means with medical imaging. Medical Imaging helps to assess the effectiveness of surgery as a treatment option; localize tumors for treatment and removal; detect the location of blood clots or other blockages; guide doctors performing joint replacements or treating fractures; and help other procedures involving the placement of devices inside the body.

Around the world, medical imaging has improved diagnoses and treatments by decreasing a significant amount of guess work done by doctors, enabling them to better deal with their patients' injuries and diseases.

1.2 Convolutional Neural Networks

Convolutional Neural Networks (CNN) is a recently popular approach to performing image recognition, which working principle is learning and concluding the characteristics from substantial input image data samples. In 1979, Japanese

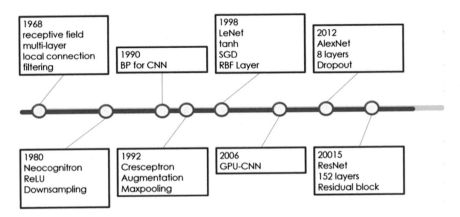

Fig. 1.2 History of the convolutional neural network

scientist Kunihiko Fukushima came up with the idea of Neocogonitron, which aimed to build a network structure that can achieve pattern recognition like the human brain and thus help us understand how the brain works [6]. In this work, he creatively introduced many new ideas from the human visual system to artificial neural networks, which nowadays are considered by many to be the prototype of CNN [5]. After the advent of LeNet5 in 1998, which was marked as the beginning of CNN, there appeared various and progressive networks, such as AlexNet 2012, VGG 2014, GoogleLeNet 2014, and ResNet 2015. The general history of CNN could be seen in Fig. 1.2.

To be more specific, similar to an actual biological neural network, CNN could identify the fraction of the image and recognize the unique feature which does not alter even if certain transformations such as shifting, scaling, and rotating. As shown in Fig. 1.3, the usual CNN consists of the following layers, Convolution layer, ReLU layer, Pooling layer, and FC (Full Connection) layer. The convolutional layer is used to extract the main features through operations. The pooling layer is very effective in reducing the size of the matrix, thus increasing efficiency. Compared with other tools of image recognition, with its own known pattern and following learning, there is no necessity to input detailed and complex mathematical arithmetic expressions for the computer to judge and CNN could come into forming specific mapping capability for further operations of detecting images.

A fully connected neural network consists of a series of fully connected layers, that connect every neuron in one layer to every neuron in the other layer. The main problem with fully connected neural networks are that the number of weights required is very large for certain types of data. For example, an image of 224 × 224 × 3 would require 150,528 weights in just the first hidden layer, and will grow quickly for even bigger images. You can imagine how computationally intensive things would become once the images reach dimensions as large as 8K resolution images (7680 × 4320), training such a network would require a lot of time and resources.

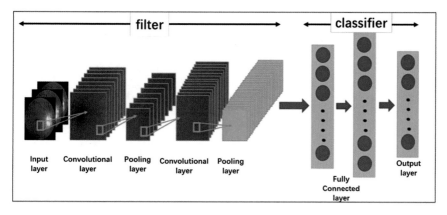

Fig. 1.3 General convolutional neural network architecture

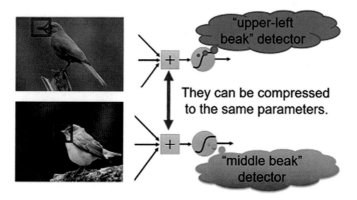

Fig. 1.4 Pattern detection in CNNs

However for image data, repeating patterns can occur in different places. Hence we can train many smaller detectors, capable of sliding across an image, to take advantage of the repeating patterns as shown in Fig. 1.4. This would reduce the number of weights required to be trained.

A Convolutional Neural Network is a neural network with some convolutional layers (and some other layers). A convolutional layer has a number of filters that does the convolutional operation (Fig. 1.5).

1.2.1 The Convolution Operation

The convolution operation shown in Fig. 1.6 is very similar to image processing filters such as the Sobel filter and Gaussian Filter. The Kernel slides across an image

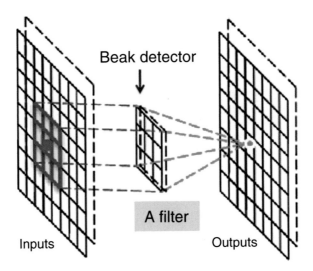

Fig. 1.5 Convolution filter

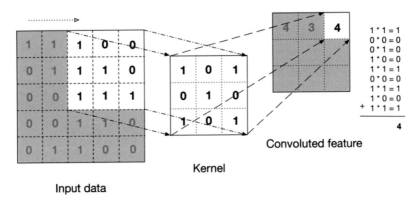

Fig. 1.6 Convolution operation

and multiplies the weights with each aligned pixel, element-wise across the filter. Afterwards the bias value is added to the output.

There are three hyperparameters deciding the spatial of the output feature map:

- Stride (S) is the step each time we slide the filter. When the stride is 1 then we move the filters one pixel at a time. When the stride is 2 (or uncommonly 3 or more, though this is rare in practice) then the filters jump 2 pixels at a time as we slide them around. This will produce smaller output volumes spatially.
- Padding (P): The inputs will be padded with a border of size according to the value specified. Most commonly, zero-padding is used to pad these locations. In neural network frameworks (caffe, tensorflow, pytorch, mxnet), the size of this

zero-padding is a hyperparameter. The size of zero-padding can also be used to control the spatial size of the output volumes.

- Depth (D): The depth of the output volume is a hyperparameter too, it corresponds to the number of filters we use for a convolution layer.

Given w as the width of input, and F is the width of the filter, with P and S as padding, the output width will be: $(W + 2P - F)/S+1$ Generally, set $P = (F - 1)/2$ when the stride is $S = 1$ ensures that the input volume and output volume will have the same size spatially.

For an input of $7 \times 7 \times 3$ and a output depth of 2, we will have 6 kernels as shown below. 3 for the first depth output and another 3 for the second depth output. The outputs of each filter is summed up to generate the output feature map.

In the example shown in Fig. 1.7, the output from each Kernel of Filter W1 is as follows:

Output of Kernel 1 = 1 Output of Kernel 2 = -2 Output of Kernel 3 = 2 Output of Filter W1 = Output of Kernel 1 + Output of Kernel 2 + Output of Kernel 3 + bias = $1 - 2 + 2 + 0 = 1$.

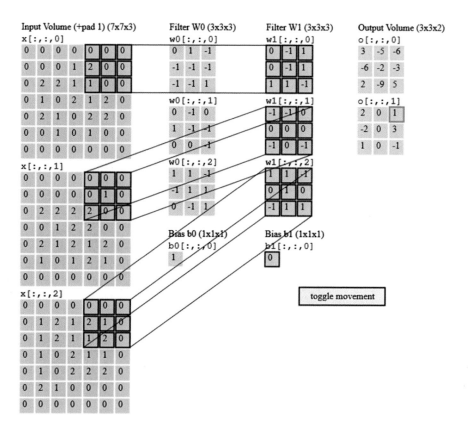

Fig. 1.7 Convolution example

Fig. 1.8 Pooling

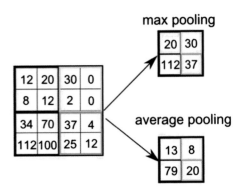

1.2.2 Pooling

Nowadays, a CNN always exploits extensive weight-sharing to reduce the degrees of the freedom of models. A pooling layer helps reduce computation time and gradually build up spatial and configural invariance. For image understanding, pooling layer helps extract more semantic meaning. The max pooling layer simply returns the maximum value over the values that the kernel operation is applied on. The example below in Fig. 1.8 illustrates the outputs of a max pooling and average pooling operation respectively, given a kernel of size 2 and stride 2.

1.2.3 Flattening

Adding a Fully-Connected layer is a (usually) cheap way of learning non-linear combinations of the high-level features as represented by the output of the convolutional layer. The Fully-Connected layer is learning a possibly non-linear function in that space.

By flattening the image into a column vector, we have converted our input image into a suitable form for our Multi-Level Perceptron. The flattened output is fed to a feed-forward neural network and backpropagation applied to every iteration of training. Over a series of epochs, the model is able to distinguish between dominating and certain low-level features in images and classify them using the Softmax Classification technique as shown in Fig. 1.9.

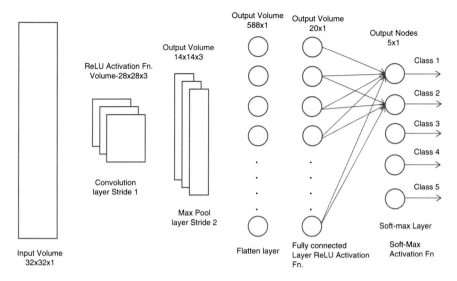

Fig. 1.9 Example of flattening

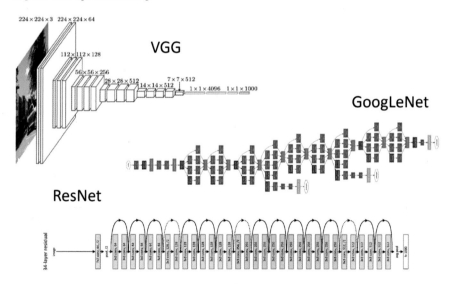

Fig. 1.10 Common CNN architectures

1.2.4 CNN Architectures

There are various network architectures being used for image classification tasks. VGG16, InceptionNet (GoogLeNet) and Resnet shown in Fig. 1.10 are some of the more notable ones.

VGG16

The VGG16 architecture garnered a lot of attention in 2014. It makes the improvement over its predecessor, AlexNet, through replacing large kernel-sized filters (11 and 5 in the first and second convolutional layer, respectively) with multiple 3×3 kernel-sized filters stacked together.

InceptionNet

before the Dense layers (which are placed at the end of the network), each time we add a new layer we face two main decisions:

1. Deciding whether we want to go with a Pooling or Convolutional operation;
2. Deciding the size and number of filters to be passed through the output of the previous layer.

Google researchers developed the Inception module allows us to apply different options all together in one single layer.

The main idea of the Inception module (in Fig. 1.11) is that of running multiple operations (pooling, convolution) with multiple filter sizes ($3 \times 3, 5 \times 5 \ldots$) in parallel so that we do not have to face any trade-off.

ResNet

Researchers thought that increasing more layers would improve the accuracy of the models. But there are two problems associated with it.

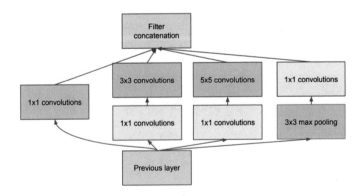

Fig. 1.11 Inception block

Fig. 1.12 Residual connections

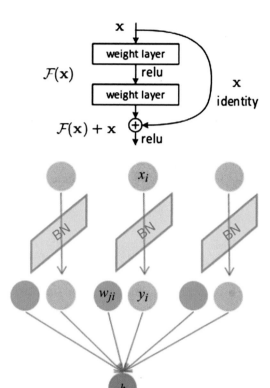

Fig. 1.13 Batch normalization

1. Vanishing gradient problem—Somewhat solved with regularization like batch normalization etc. Gradients become increasingly smaller as the network becomes deeper, making it harder to train deep networks.
2. The authors observed that adding more layers didn't improve the accuracy. Also, it is not over-fitting also as the training error is also increasing.

The basic intuition of the Residual connections (Fig. 1.12) is that, at each conv layer the network learns some features about the data $F(x)$ and passes the remaining errors further into the network. So we can say the output error of the conv layer is $H(x) = F(x) - x$.

This solution also helped to alleviate the vanishing gradient problem as gradients can flow through the residual connections.

ResNet also utilized batch normalization to reduce the effects of the internal covariate shift. This normalization is carried out for a single neuron. It uses the data of a mini-batch during network training to calculate the mean and variance of the neuron, so it is called batch normalization. The general process could be seen in Fig. 1.13.

Through the following transformation equations shown, we solved the first problem by normalizing the data in a more simplified way, so that the distribution mean of each feature of the input of the first layer is 0 and the variance is 1.

$$\mu_i = \frac{1}{M} \sum x_i$$

$$\sigma_i = \sqrt{\frac{1}{M} \sum (x_i - \mu_i)^2 + \epsilon}$$

As mentioned above, Normalization mitigates internal covariate shift issues by stabilizing the distribution of input data across each layer of the network, but it leads to a loss of data representation. In other words, we change the representation ability of the network of the original data through transformation operations, so that the parameter information learned by the underlying network is lost. On the other hand, by making the mean and variance of the input distribution of each layer equal to 0, the input is easy to fall into the linear region of the nonlinear activation function when it passes through the sigmoid or tanh activation function. This alleviates the gradient disappearance problem. Therefore, Batch Normalization introduces two learnable parameters γ and β. The introduction of these two parameters is to restore the expression ability of the data itself and perform a linear transformation on normalized data, namely. In particular, when can realize identity transform and retain distribution information of original input features. At the same time, Batch Normalization makes the model less sensitive to the parameters in the network, simplifies the parameter tuning process, and makes the network learning more stable.

Through the above steps, we can ensure the expressiveness of the input data to a certain extent.

Batch Normalization makes each network layer of the input data of the mean and variance are all within a certain range by standardization and linear transformation. The latter layer network does not need to constantly adapt to the changes in the input of the bottom network, thus realizing the decoupling between the middle layer and the layer of the network. In addition, it allows each layer to learn independently, which is conducive to improving the learning speed of the whole neural network.

1.2.5 Finetuning

Neural networks are usually initialized with random weights. these weights will converge to some values after training for a series of epochs, to allow us to properly classify our input images. However, instead of a random initialization, we can initialize those weights to values that are already good to classify a different dataset.

Transfer Learning is the process of training a network that already performs well on one task, to perform a different task. Finetuning is an example of transfer learning, where we use another network trained on a much larger dataset to initialize and simply train it for classification. In finetuning, We can keep the weights of earlier layers as it has been observed that the Early layers contain more generic features, edges, color blobs and are more common to many visual tasks. Thus we can just Fine-tune the later layers which are more specific to the details of the class.

Through Transfer Learning, We would not require a dataset as big compared to having to train a network from scratch. We can reduce the required number of images from hundreds of thousands or even millions of images down to just a few thousands. Training Time is also sped up during the retraining process as it is much easier due to the initialization.

1.3 Data Augmentation

More training data often leads to an increase in a deep learning model's performance. By introducing slight alterations to the training instances, the approach of "data augmentation" adds more photos to the training set [8]. It is a well-known and widely used technique for computer vision problems. It lets you create new training instances that belong to the same class as the underlying instance. The trained model is more robust and more generalizable thanks to data augmentation. The original data is perturbed randomly using a wide range of approaches.

Translations, distortions, flips (horizontal and vertical), brightness adjustments, scale adjustments, ZCA and PCA whitening are some examples of frequently used augmentations.

When data augmentation is used, each epoch the network sees a slightly different image. In most cases, data augmentation is only used during training and not testing.

The increase in data variety leads to less overfitting and better accuracy performance. Data augmentation has the ability to significantly enhance model accuracy, especially on tiny datasets like 17-flowers (Fig. 1.14).

1.4 Regularization

One of the most important components of training your machine learning model is avoiding overfitting [4]. If the model is overfitting, its accuracy will be low. This occurs as a result of your model attempting to capture the noise in your training dataset. When we refer to "noise," we mean the data points that just reflect random chance rather than the inherent characteristics of your data. Your model becomes more adaptive as a result of learning such data points, but at the cost of overfitting.

In this type of regression, the coefficient estimates are constrained, regularized, or shrunk in the direction of zero. To minimize overfitting, this strategy inhibits learning more sophisticated or flexible models.

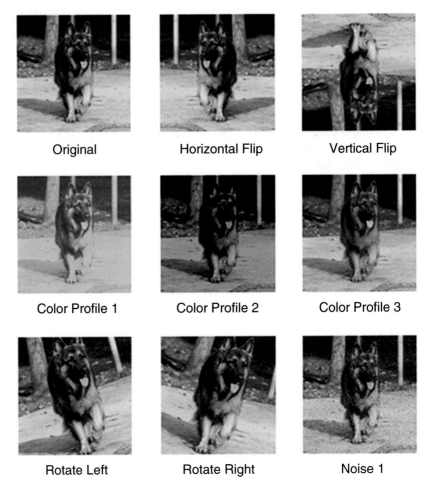

Fig. 1.14 Examples of data augmentations

This is an illustration of a straightforward linear regression relationship. Here, Y stands for the learnt relationship and β for the coefficient estimates for various predictors or variables (X).

$$Y \approx \beta 0 + \beta 1 X 1 + \beta 2 X 2 + \ldots + \beta p X p$$

A loss function called the residual sum of squares, or RSS, is used throughout the fitting process. The coefficients are selected to minimize RSS.

$$RSS = \sum_{i=1}^{n} (y_i - \beta_0 - \sum_{j=1}^{p} \beta_j x_{ij})^2$$

This will now modify the coefficients in accordance with your training data. The computed coefficients won't generalize well to the subsequent data if there is noise in the training data. Regularization steps in at this point and reduces or regularizes these learnt estimates in the direction of zero.

1.4.1 Ridge Regression

$$\sum_{i=1}^{n}(y_i - \beta_0 - \sum_{j=1}^{p}\beta_j x_{ij})^2 + \lambda\sum_{j=1}^{p}\beta_j^2 = RSS + \lambda\sum_{j=1}^{p}\beta_j^2$$

Ridge regression is a type of linear regression in which we add a small amount of bias, called the Ridge regression penalty, so that we can make better predictions [3]. The L2-norm is another name for it.

In this method, the cost function is modified by adding a penalty term (shrinkage term) that multiplies lambda by the squared weight of each feature.

The usage of conventional linear or polynomial regression will not work when the independent variables have a significant degree of collinearity (problem of multicollinearity), hence Ridge regression can be employed to address these issues.

In the event that there are more parameters than there are samples, using Ridge regression can also assist to resolve the problems.

1.4.2 Lasso Regression

$$\sum_{i=1}^{n}(y_i - \beta_0 - \sum_{j=1}^{p}\beta_j x_{ij})^2 + \lambda\sum_{j=1}^{p}|\beta_j| = RSS + \lambda\sum_{j=1}^{p}|\beta_j|$$

Another variation of the regularization approach used to lessen the model's complexity is lasso regression [3]. It is often referred to as the L1-norm and stands for Least Absolute and Selection Operator.

The only difference between it and the Ridge Regression is that the penalty term now includes the absolute weights rather than a square of weights.

When the tuning parameter λ is big enough, the L1 penalty has the effect of driving some of the coefficient estimations to exactly equal zero, which completely eliminates some characteristics for model evaluation. As a result, the lasso approach is believed to produce sparse models and also conducts feature selection.

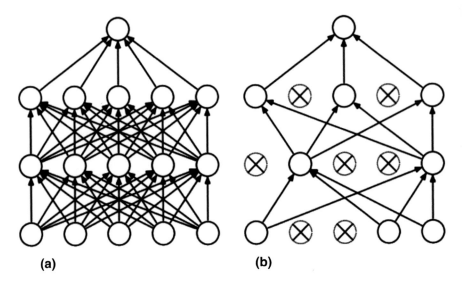

Fig. 1.15 Dropout. (**a**) Standard neural net. (**b**) After applying dropout

1.4.3 Dropout

A regularization technique called dropout (Fig. 1.15) mimics training an enormous number of neural networks with various topologies concurrently [1].

During training, certain layer outputs are disregarded or "dropped out" at random. As a result, the layer has fewer nodes and edges than the preceding layer and is considered as such. This results in layer updates being conducted with a different configuration during training.

As a result of dropout, the training becomes noisy, causing the nodes in a layer to probabilistically increase or reduce their responsibility for the inputs.

This approach implies that dropout is likely to break apart scenarios in which network levels co-adapt to correct for errors in earlier layers, hence boosting the model's resilience.

It works with the majority of layer types, including convolutional layers, recurrent layers, and dense fully connected layers.

In implementation, a new hyperparameter is added that specifies the likelihood of the layer's outputs being dropped out. Another possibility is that the hyperparameter could define the percentage of the layer's outputs that will be retained.

After training is complete, dropout is not utilized in the inferencing of the trained network.

Dropout will cause the network's weights to scale up. As a result, in order to finalize the network, the weights are first transformed such that they are scaled according to the selected dropout rate. The network may then be utilized to make predictions as usual after completion.

References

1. Brownlee, J. (2019). A gentle introduction to dropout for regularizing deep neural networks.
2. Brush, K. (2019). What is medical imaging?
3. Goyal, C. (2021). Regularization: Regularization techniques in machine learning.
4. Gupta, P. (2017). Regularization in machine learning.
5. He, K., Zhang, X., Ren, S., & Sun, J. (2015). Deep residual learning for image recognition. CoRR. abs/1512.03385.
6. Kolla, M., & Venugopal, T. (2021). Efficient classification of diabetic retinopathy using binary cnn. In *2021 International conference on computational intelligence and knowledge economy (ICCIKE)* (pp. 244–247).
7. Lecun, Y., Bottou, L., Bengio, Y., & Haffner, P. (1998). Gradient-based learning applied to document recognition. *Proceedings of the IEEE, 86*(11), 2278–2324.
8. Robinet, L. (2020). Data augmentation and handling huge datasets with keras: A simple way.

Chapter 2
CNN for Brain Tumor Classification

2.1 Introduction to Brain Tumors

In both children and adults, brain tumors are regarded as one of the most aggressive disorders. Brain tumors are the main diagnosis for around 85% of all Central Nervous System (CNS) malignancies [10]. Each year, doctors identify 11,700 patients with brain tumors. The likelihood of survival for women with a malignant brain or CNS tumor is around 36% in the following 5 years, while the chance for males is even lower, at 34%.

There are two categories of tumors: benign and malignant.

2.1.1 Benign Tumors

Benign tumors are tumors that do not spread to other parts of the body and remain in their original position. Typically, benign tumors develop slowly and have identifiable boundaries [9].

Benign tumors often do not cause any problems. However, there is a chance that these tumors might enlarge and apply pressure on surrounding tissues, resulting in discomfort or other health issues [9]. For instance, a big benign lung tumor might continue to expand and compress the trachea, making breathing difficult. Such situations would call for an immediate surgical removal. Benign tumors are unlikely to recur after removal. Fibroids in the uterus and lipomas in the skin are two examples of benign tumors.

© The Author(s), under exclusive license to Springer Nature Singapore Pte Ltd. 2023
T. T. Teoh, *Convolutional Neural Networks for Medical Applications*, SpringerBriefs in Computer Science, https://doi.org/10.1007/978-981-19-8814-1_2

2.1.2 Malignant Tumors

On the other hand, malignant tumors include cells that would spread locally and/or to distant places and develop uncontrolled. As a result, malignant tumors are regarded as cancerous because they spread to distant areas through the lymphatic or blood systems [9]. Metastasis refers to this process of spreading. The liver, lungs, brain, and bone are the most frequently affected organs by metastasis, although it can happen anywhere in the body.

To stop malignant tumors from spreading, treatment is necessary. If discovered early, surgery is usually the suggested course of treatment, with chemotherapy or radiation as backup options. The suggested course of treatment is likely to be systemic, such as chemotherapy or immunotherapy, if the disease has already spread to other bodily regions [9].

Some benign tumors may develop into malignant tumors in the future. It may be necessary to have surgery to remove these tumors, thus they need to be carefully watched. For instance, colon polyps, another term for an abnormal clump of cells, can develop into cancer and are often removed surgically.

In order to increase the life expectancy of the patients, appropriate therapy, careful planning, and precise diagnostics should be carried out. Magnetic Resonance Imaging (MRI) is the most effective method for finding brain cancers. The scans provide an enormous quantity of image data, which would be examined by a radiologist. Because of the complexity of brain tumors and their characteristics, a manual examination might be prone to mistakes.

Application of automated classification techniques using Machine Learning and Artificial Intelligence has consistently shown higher accuracy than manual classification. Hence, proposing a system performing detection and classification by using Deep Learning Algorithms using Convolutional Neural Network (CNN) would be helpful to doctors all around the world.

2.2   Brain Tumor Dataset

In this dataset, we have a total of 3264 images. These images are classified into 4 different classes, namely no tumor, glioma tumor, meningioma tumor and pituitary tumor [10].

Each year in the United States, about 20,000 people are newly diagnosed with gliomas, 170,000 people are diagnosed with meningioma and 10,000 are diagnosed with pituitary tumors [10].

2.2.1 Glioma Tumor

A glioma is a tumor that develops when glial cells proliferate uncontrollably [1]. Under normal circumstances, these cells serve as a support for nerves and contribute to the proper functioning of your central nervous system. Most of the time, gliomas grow in the brain, but they can also grow in the spinal cord.

Although gliomas are malignant, some of them seem to proliferate extremely slowly. Mostly, they are brain tumors that have their origins in the brain. Although gliomas typically only affect the brain and spine, they are dangerous because they may spread to other parts of the brain that are difficult to access and treat surgically.

Gliomas may be divided into three primary categories depending on the kind of glial cell that they originate from. Mixed gliomas are a subcategory of these tumors that may have numerous cell types present. Based on its development rate and other characteristics, healthcare professionals would categorize each form of glioma as low-, mid-, or high-grade.

Gliomas include:

- Astrocytomas: These tumors develop from astrocytes, a type of glial cell. In adults, the most common type of malignant brain tumor is an astrocytoma. They are the most prevalent kind of glioma seen in children. Glioblastomas are the name for aggressive or quickly growing astrocytomas. Diffuse intrinsic pontine gliomas (DIPGs) are an uncommon but extremely aggressive kind of brain cancer in children. It mostly affects youngsters and develops in the brain stem.
- Ependymomas: Ependymomas are tumors that start in ependymocytes, which are glial cells. Ependymomas typically form in the spinal cord or brain ventricles. Although they might spread through the cerebrospinal fluid, which surrounds the brain and spinal cord as protection, these tumors do not invade other parts of the body than the brain or spine. Ependymomas make for around 2% of all brain tumors. Children seem to get it more frequently than adults do.
- Oligodendrogliomas: These tumors develop from oligodendrocytes, which are glial cells. Although oligodendrogliomas typically expand slowly, they may eventually become more aggressive. Oligodendrogliomas, like epidermoid tumors, seldom metastasize outside of the brain or spine. Adults are more likely to have them than youngsters. Oligodendrogliomas account for 1–2% of all brain tumors.

Who Does it Affect

Gliomas are more frequently discovered in children (under 12) and elderly people (over 65). Gliomas may affect white people more frequently than other races. The chance of developing gliomas might possibly rise if you have certain inherited genetic diseases. Men are somewhat more likely than women to get gliomas. Long-term or repeated exposure to radiation or certain chemicals may raise your risk. With low-grade or slow-growing gliomas, young patients have the best prognosis.

Survival Rates

Glioma survival rates vary depending on the patient's age, tumor variety, and grade. The prognosis may also be impacted by certain mutations. The outlook gets worse the older someone is when they are diagnosed and start treatment. Survival rates are greatest in adults and children for low-grade ependymomas, oligodendrogliomas, and astrocytomas. Glioblastomas, have the lowest (between 6 and 20%).

Complications

Complications of gliomas include:

- Brain hemorrhage.
- Brain herniation.
- Hydrocephalus.
- Internal pressure within your skull.
- Seizures.

2.2.2 Meningioma Tumor

A meningioma is a tumor that develops in the three layers of tissue that surround and shield your brain and spinal cord, known as the meninges [2]. The most frequent form of tumor to develop in the head is a meningioma. These tumors may compress or pressure nearby brain tissue, nerves, or blood arteries, which might be dangerous.

Although meningiomas often are benign tumors, occasionally they can also be cancerous. The majority of meningiomas develop slowly, frequently over several years, and seldom cause symptoms. They are frequently only discovered until they have become fairly huge. Meningiomas can occasionally result in severe handicap and even pose a threat to your life if they compress and impact your brain's adjacent locations. They typically do not need urgent treatment because of their slow development and are watched over time.

By grade, there are three different meningioma types:

- Grade I or typical: This benign meningioma is slow-growing. Eighty percent of instances fit this description.
- Grade II or atypical: This benign meningioma develops quicker and might be harder to cure. Grade II instances make about 17% of all cases.
- Grade III or anaplastic: This meningioma is malignant (cancerous), has rapid growth, and spreads fast. These tumors account for around 1.7% of cases.

Meningiomas can vary in kind depending on where they are located and what kind of tissue they are made of. Examples of places include:

- Convexity meningiomas, which develop on the surface of the brain and which, as they develop, may put pressure on the brain.
- Intraventricular meningiomas, which develop inside the brain's ventricles. Cerebrospinal fluid (CSF) is transported through these ventricles.
- Olfactory groove meningiomas are found near the base of the skull, between the brain and the nose. They develop close to the olfactory nerve, which controls your sense of smell.
- Sphenoid wing meningiomas, which manifest themselves along a bony ridge behind your eyes.

Who Does it Affect

Meningiomas can still occur in kids, although they are significantly more prevalent in adults. Since the typical age of diagnosis is 66 years old, they are frequently seen when people are older. Meningioma seems to affect black individuals more frequently than other ethnic groups in the US.

Meningiomas are more common in females than in males. This is probably caused by hormonal elements that have a role in meningioma growth. However, males are more likely than females to develop malignant meningiomas.

Survival Rates

The following variables affect the meningioma prognosis:

- The size of the tumor.
- The location of the tumor.
- If the tumor is benign or malignant.
- Whether surgery could be used to completely or partially remove the tumor.
- Your age and general health.

One of the best indicators of the prognosis for adults, is their age upon diagnosis. Your outlook seems to be better in general the younger you are. Complete tumor removal improves results, but isn't always feasible due to tumor position.

Meningiomas are capable of returning even after therapy (recur). The degree of surgical excision affects the meningioma's propensity to return. Lower recurrence rates are linked to complete surgical removal.

Complications

Meningiomas and their treatments can result in long-term issues [8], such as:

- Difficulty concentrating
- Loss of memory

- Personality changes
- Seizures
- Weakness
- Language difficulties

2.2.3 Pituitary Tumor

At the base of the brain, there is a small gland called the pituitary gland that is about the size of a pea. As the body's "master gland," it creates and stores a wide variety of hormones that circulate throughout the body, regulating various bodily functions or inducing the production of more hormones in other glands [3].

Tumors of the pituitary gland are abnormal growths that form there. The majority of pituitary tumors are benign. They typically remain in the tissues around the pituitary gland or in that region, and they are unlikely to travel to other areas of your body. Pituary tumors come in two varieties: functional and nonfunctional. Non-functional tumors inhibit the production of hormones, whereas functioning tumors produce an excessive amount of a hormone that is normally produced by the pituitary gland. Both kinds may develop problems if they are big and obstruct the pituitary gland's ability to operate, or put pressure on nearby brain areas.

Functioning pituitary tumors overproduce a hormone that the pituitary gland typically produces. The diseases brought on by functioning pituitary tumors include:

- Prolactinoma
- Acromegaly and gigantism
- Cushing's Disease
- Thyroid stimulating hormone (TSH)-secreting tumors

The three most prevalent forms of non-functioning tumors are Rathke's cleft cysts, craniopharyngiomas, and non-functioning pituitary adenomas. The pituitary region can also have tumors of different kind. Most of which don't have cancer. Other disorders that can affect the pituitary, such inflammation and infections, may be mistaken for tumors on MRI scans.

Who Does it Affect

Ten to fifteen percent of all tumors that form inside the skull are pituitary adenomas. It's estimated that up to 20% of people actually experience them at some time throughout their life. However, a lot of pituitary adenomas, particularly microadenomas, don't manifest any symptoms at all and go undetected. In comparison to microadenomas, macroroadenomas are nearly twice as common. Though they can develop at any age, pituitary adenomas are more likely among persons in their 30s and 40s. People younger than 20 rarely have them. Adenomas are more common in women than in men.

Survival Rates

Pituitary tumors can be treated in a variety of ways, such as by surgically removing the tumor, limiting its development, and adjusting your hormone levels with medicine. The doctor might advise continuing to keep an eye on its growth.

Dopamine agonist medications are often effective in treating prolactinoma, a functioning pituitary tumor. This medicine should eliminate or decrease symptoms, drop prolactin levels to normal, repair pituitary function, and shrink tumor size.

Symptoms

Symptoms aren't always present with pituitary tumors. Sometimes, they are unintentionally picked up during an imaging examination like an MRI or CT that was conducted for a different cause. Depending on the hormone they produce, functioning pituitary tumors can trigger a range of symptoms. Signs and symptoms of nonfunctioning pituitary tumors are frequently tied to the development of the tumors themselves and the pressure that they impose on surrounding tissues.

Macroadenomas are massive pituitary tumors that are 1 centimeter (slightly less than half an inch) or bigger. Microadenomas, on the other hand, are tiny tumors. Due to their size, macroadenomas can push on the pituitary and surrounding structures.

Due to their size, macroadenomas can push on the pituitary and surrounding structures.

Complications

Blindness is among the most harmful side effects. It might occur if a tumor places an undue amount of pressure on your optic nerves, which are situated near to your pituitary gland. However, not every person with a pituitary tumor will experience visual issues. In most cases, tumor development and eyesight loss occur quite gradually.

pituitary apoplexy: A uncommon yet dangerous condition that involves unexpected bleeding into the pituitary tumor.

permanent hormone deficiency: Pituitary tumors may cause a permanent imbalance of hormones.

diabetes insipidus: Unlike type 1 or type 2 diabetes, this illness results in a rise in blood glucose levels and is typically linked to bigger pituitary tumors.

2.3   Classifying Brain Tumors

Brain Tumors are complex as there can be a lot of abnormalities in their sizes and location. Thus it is very challenging to gain a complete understanding of the tumor. Furthermore, MRIs of these tumors require professional Neurosurgeons to analyse them. Developing countries generally lack skillful doctors and knowledge about brain tumors. This makes it really challenging and time-consuming to generate reports from MRIs. Automated brain tumor classification using CNNs could potentially help alleviate these issues.

In many cases, data is easy to obtain, and in the case of 2D images, scanning or picture-shooting is very common and applicable. Brain tumors from CT scans can be collected and annotated accordingly. Thus, Convolution Neural Nets can be developed to classify brain tumors.

However, data processing of these images can be very cumbersome and difficult. Images collected from CT scans in our Brain Tumor dataset have to be processed into a form suitable for computer calculations. Furthermore, in order to improve the predictive capabilities of the neural network on such data, specific image enhancements have to be applied on them. This way, certain key features could be enhanced and other irrelevant features would be mitigated. This allows the model obtained from training to have a stronger generalization ability, improved ability to resist noise, and reduce the likelihood of overfitting[11, 12].

Thus we use three different data augmentation methods for model overfitting: traditional flip augmentation, RandomColor augmentation, and mixup augmentation. Flip enhancement can freely flip the picture, play the role of position transformation of input information and enhance the adaptability of the model to the subtle transformation of samples. The RandomColor enhancement can randomly adjust the color of the image, highlight the lesion information to a certain extent, and make it easier for the model to learn key features. The mixup method is different from the traditional data enhancement method which was proposed in 2018 [12]. It is a simple and data-independent data enhancement method. Mixup models the domain relationship between different samples of different classes, and trains on virtual samples (that is, constructed as a linear interpolation of two random samples in the training set and their labels) [12]. Mixup helps to eliminate memory for mislabels and sensitivity to adversarial examples. Stabilities in adversarial training can be improved as well [12].

These methods are used to train a custom convolutional neural network and we will compare its performance against a base model without data augmentation.

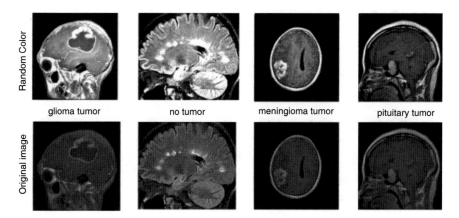

Fig. 2.1 Examples of RandomColor method

2.3.1   Data Augmentation Method

RandomColor

RandomColor is a method to adjust the color of an image by setting random saturation, brightness, contrast, and sharpness of this image. This method is achieved by the related functions of the ImageEnhance module called from the PIL module. Besides, the random number generated by the random() function in the numpy module. The effect of images is as follows (Fig. 2.1):

Flip or Rotation

The second method is Flip or Rotation. The method adopted in this paper is that 50% of the MRI images are processed by horizontal flipping, and the remaining half are rotated by random angles. In the experiment, the horizontal flip is achieved by setting the transpose function parameter in the Image module in the PIL module to 'FLIP_LEFT_RIGHT'. Meanwhile, the random function in the numpy module is called to generate a random angle as the parameter of the rotate function. These two methods are commonly used methods for medical image data enhancement. In this paper, these two methods are synthesized in proportion for data enhancement. In Fig. 2.2, we show some examples of this method

Mixup

Mixup is utilized in preprocessing for MRI images in our last experiment, which can improve the robustness of our image dataset[12]. This data augmentation is

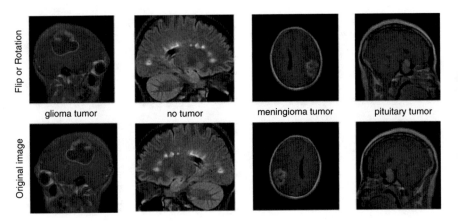

Fig. 2.2 Examples of flip or rotation method

glioma tumor : label: 0 → one-hot encoding: [1. 0. 0. 0. 0. 0. 0. 0. 0. 0.]

no tumor : label: 1 → one-hot encoding: [0. 1. 0. 0. 0. 0. 0. 0. 0. 0.]

meningioma tumor : label: 2 → one-hot encoding: [0. 0. 1. 0. 0. 0. 0. 0. 0. 0.]

pituitary tumor : label: 3 → one-hot encoding: [0. 0. 0. 1. 0. 0. 0. 0. 0. 0.]

Fig. 2.3 Examples of one-hot encoding

essentially a generic vicinal distribution[12]:

$$\mu(\tilde{x}, \tilde{y}|x_i, y_i) = \frac{1}{n} \sum_{j}^{n} \mathbb{E}_\lambda[\delta(\tilde{x} = \lambda \cdot x_i + (1 - \lambda) \cdot x_j, \tilde{y} = \lambda \cdot y_i + (1 - \lambda) \cdot y_j)]$$

In this distribution equation, x_i is the input image and y_i is the relative label of x_i. $\tilde{x}$ and $\tilde{y}$ are new input image and label generated from x_i and y_i. $\lambda \sim \text{Beta}(\alpha, \alpha)$ where $\alpha \in (0, \infty)$. According to this distribution the relationship between xi and $\tilde{x}$, y_i and $\tilde{y}$ can be represented by:

$$\tilde{x} = \lambda x_i + (1 - \lambda)x_j,$$

$$\tilde{y} = \lambda y_i + (1 - \lambda)y_j$$

In our experiment, the value of alpha was set to be 0.8 which is a new value setting, and mixup generated new dataset by combine two randomly images in different categories, which can fuse features from two images. Meanwhile, the labels also are combined. As shown in the equation the relationships between them are linearly proportional. Labels were turned to be 10 bit one-hot encoding, which can handle discrete features as shown in Fig. 2.3.

There were several functions called from numpy used to achieve the algorithm before. The effect of this enhancement is shown (Fig. 2.4):

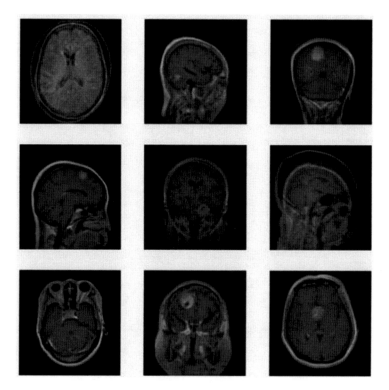

Fig. 2.4 Examples of mixup method

2.3.2 Convolution and Pooling Layers

max pooling layers. In convolutional layers, we all used 3 × 3 filters, and the parameters of padding was set to be "same", so there is no loss of image feature. Besides, the max pooling layers are downsized feature map to the half of input. Dropout[5] and Batch Normalization[6] were used to reduce the effect of overfitting.

Especially, the global average pooling layer, proposed in[7], replace fully connected layers and can effectively solve the overfitting problem by reducing the amounts of parameters (Fig. 2.5).

2.3.3 Global Average Pooling (GAP)

We utilized the GAP layer as the output layer. If the last feature shape is 8 × 8 × 128, GAP can calculate the average values on each channel to produce a 1D vector with length 128. This vector will then be fed directly to the output layer instead of going through a fully connected layer (Fig. 2.6).

Fig. 2.5 The structure of the neural network

```
Model: "sequential"

 Layer (type)                 Output Shape              Param #
=================================================================
 conv2d (Conv2D)              (None, 256, 256, 16)      448

 batch_normalization (BatchN  (None, 256, 256, 16)      64
 ormalization)

 max_pooling2d (MaxPooling2D  (None, 128, 128, 16)      0
 )

 dropout (Dropout)            (None, 128, 128, 16)      0

 conv2d_1 (Conv2D)            (None, 128, 128, 32)      4640

 batch_normalization_1 (Batc  (None, 128, 128, 32)      128
 hNormalization)

 max_pooling2d_1 (MaxPooling  (None, 64, 64, 32)        0
 2D)

 dropout_1 (Dropout)          (None, 64, 64, 32)        0

 conv2d_2 (Conv2D)            (None, 64, 64, 64)        18496

 batch_normalization_2 (Batc  (None, 64, 64, 64)        256
 hNormalization)

 max_pooling2d_2 (MaxPooling  (None, 32, 32, 64)        0
 2D)

 dropout_2 (Dropout)          (None, 32, 32, 64)        0

 conv2d_3 (Conv2D)            (None, 32, 32, 128)       73856

 batch_normalization_3 (Batc  (None, 32, 32, 128)       512
 hNormalization)

 max_pooling2d_3 (MaxPooling  (None, 16, 16, 128)       0
 2D)

 dropout_3 (Dropout)          (None, 16, 16, 128)       0

 conv2d_4 (Conv2D)            (None, 16, 16, 512)       590336

 batch_normalization_4 (Batc  (None, 16, 16, 512)       2048
 hNormalization)

 max_pooling2d_4 (MaxPooling  (None, 8, 8, 512)         0
 2D)

 global_average_pooling2d (G  (None, 512)               0
 lobalAveragePooling2D)

 dense (Dense)                (None, 10)                5130

=================================================================
Total params: 695,914
Trainable params: 694,410
Non-trainable params: 1,504
```

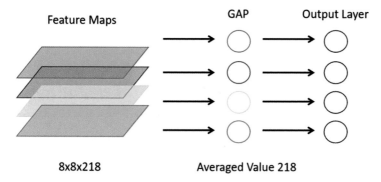

Fig. 2.6 The structure of the GAP method

In our experiments, we used 3 functions: EarlyStopping, ModelCheckpoint, and ReduceLROnPlateau called from callbacks module in keras to stop training early to reduce overfitting, save the best model during the training, and reduce the learning rate to achieve higher accuracy.

2.3.4 Training

To compare between the impacts of the different augmentation methods, we trained 4 separate CNN models utilizing different image enhancement operations: RandomColor, Flip or Rotation and mixup and without image enhancement. We split the brain tumor MRI dataset into train data, validation data and test data. The train set was processed with different enhancement methods. The training epoch were all set to 100 so that all models were able to converge. The models were then trained on the different train sets and we plot out the loss and accuracy of the validation sets. Finally, we determine the performance of our models on test set.

2.3.5 Result

From these figures, it can be seen that on the Fig. 2.7, the training data after RandomColor enhancement performed even worse than the train set without image enhancement. It proved that RandomColor is not suitable to use in this brain tumor dataset (Table 2.1). Although this enhancement had good performance on the training set with a fast fitting speed, it cannot perform well on the validation set.

On the Fig. 2.8, it could be seen that the Flip or Rotation can slow down the fitting speed in training and did better in validation set than the training set without enhancement. It can reduce the effect of overfitting and the second picture in Fig. 2.8 shows the trend of loss function of Flip or Rotation will be lower than the loss of

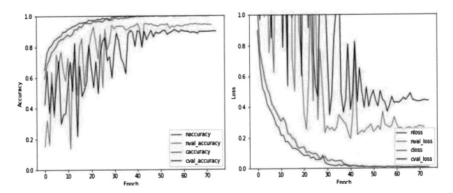

Fig. 2.7 Training and validation: Accuracy curve (left) and Loss curve (right) RandomColor(c) vs Without enhancement(n)

Table 2.1 Train accuracy (100 epochs) and best Test accuracy

	Without	RandomColor	Flip or Rotation	mixup
Train	1.0	1.0	0.9996	0.962
Test	0.903	0.817	0.921	0.947

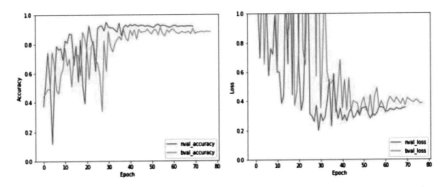

Fig. 2.8 Validation: Accuracy curve (left) and loss curve (right) Flip or Rotation(b) vs without enhancement(n)

without enhancement. It was proved that the Flip and Rotation can effectively reduce the loss of test set.

It is shown that the mixup training set loss was lower than the Flip or Rotation and validation accuracy was almost the same in Fig. 2.9. In summary, mixup performed better than the Flip or Rotation in training model. It was proved that mixup can effectively handle the overfitting problem. Consider the accuracy on train set after running 100 times of epoch, train set without enhancement reaches 100%, RandomColor reaches 100%, Flip or Rotation reaches 99.96% and mixup reaches 96.2%. Consider the best accuracy on test set, model without enhancement reaches 90.3%, RandomColor reaches 81.7%, Flip or Rotation reaches 92.1% and mixup reaches 94.7%. This result is consistent with these three comparison figures, that is,

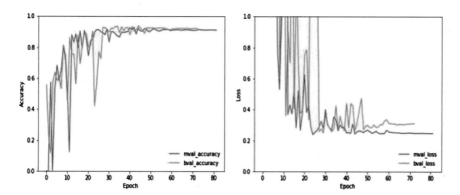

Fig. 2.9 Validation: Accuracy curve (left) and loss curve (right) mixup(m) vs Flip or Rotation(b)

mixup is the best in reducing overfitting, Flip or Rotation also has good robustness capacity, but RandomColor even aggravates overfitting problem.

2.3.6 Conclusion

In conclusion, we compare the image enhancement called mixup with other fundamental image enhancement: RandomColor and Flip or Rotation on the brain tumor MRI dataset. In order to illustrate the usefulness of mixup in brain tumor classification, we compared the results of training without enhancement, using RandomColor, Flip or Rotation and mixup. The results showed that models were able to achieve an accuracy of 90.3%, 81.7%, 92.1%, and 94.7% respectively on the test set [4]. Mixup uses images of train set in different categories in combination to generate a new train set, which makes the trained CNN more robust, thereby effectively reducing the likelihood of overfitting. Comparing against the other two methods, it shows better performance in the classification of brain tumor MRI. Hence, a CNN trained with mixup will be suitable for developing a brain tumor classssifier to help identify the presence and type of brain tumor from MRI Images.

References

1. Cleveland Clinic. (2021). Glioma: What is it, causes, symptoms, treatment and; outlook.
2. Cleveland Clinic. (2022). Meningioma: What it is, causes, symptoms and treatment.
3. Cleveland Clinic. (2022). Pituitary adenomas: Definition, symptoms and treatment.
4. Du, Y., Chen, Z., & Teoh, T. T. (2022). Effect of mixup enhancement on cnn network for brain tumor classification. In *2022 Asia conference on cloud computing, computer vision and image processing (3CVIP)*.

5. Hinton, G. E., Srivastava, N., Krizhevsky, A., Sutskever, I., & Salakhutdinov, R. (2012). Improving neural networks by preventing co-adaptation of feature detectors. *CoRR*, abs/1207.0580.
6. Ioffe, S., & Szegedy, C. (2015). Batch normalization: Accelerating deep network training by reducing internal covariate shift. *CoRR*, abs/1502.03167.
7. Lin, M., Chen, Q., & Yan, S. (2013). Network in network. arxiv:1312.4400. Comment: 10 pages, 4 figures, for iclr2014.
8. Mayo Clinic. (2022). Meningioma.
9. Patel, A. (2020). Benign vs malignant tumors.
10. Sartaj, B. (2020). Brain tumor classification (mri).
11. Shijie, J., Ping, W., Peiyi, J., & Siping, H. (2017). Research on data augmentation for image classification based on convolution neural networks. In *2017 chinese automation congress (CAC)* (pp. 4165–4170).
12. Zhang, H., Cissé, M., Dauphin, Y. N., & Lopez-Paz, D. (2017). Mixup: Beyond empirical risk minimization. *CoRR*, abs/1710.09412.

Chapter 3
CNN for Pneumonia Image Classification

3.1 Introduction to Pneumonia

On a global scale, pneumonia is one of the leading causes of mortality. People who have other significant, persistent conditions often succumb to pneumonia as the last sickness before passing away. Each year, over 4–5 million Americans contract pneumonia, and 55,000 of individuals pass away [9]. Pneumonia is the most common infectious cause of mortality in the United States, ranking eighth overall along with influenza. Pneumonia is the leading cause of mortality among illnesses that develop while patients are hospitalized, as well as the leading cause of death overall in underdeveloped nations. With an annual incidence of 34–40 cases per 1000 children in Europe and North America, pneumonia is also one of the most prevalent severe illnesses among kids and babies [9].

3.1.1 Causes of Pneumonia

Different microbes, such as bacteria, viruses, mycobacteria, fungus, and parasites, can cause pneumonia. Mycobacterial, fungal, and parasite pneumonias are far less prevalent than bacterial and viral pneumonias. Depending on the person's age, health, location, and other conditions, different organisms may be present. There also might be multiple microorganisms at play. For instance, bacterial pneumonia frequently causes influenza (a viral infection) to be more difficult to treat.

T. T. Teoh, *Convolutional Neural Networks for Medical Applications*, SpringerBriefs in Computer Science, https://doi.org/10.1007/978-981-19-8814-1_3

3.1.2 Categories of Pneumonia

Pneumonia comes in more than 30 distinct types, which are categorized according to their causes [4]. The most common kinds of pneumonia include:

- Bacterial pneumonia. Several types of bacteria cause this type of pneumonia. Streptococcus pneumonia is the most pervasive. It typically happens when the body is compromised in some manner, such as through disease, inadequate nutrition, aging, or decreased immunity, allowing the germs to enter the lungs.
- Bacterial pneumonia can strike people of any age, but it is more likely to happen if you misuse alcohol, smoke cigarettes, are elderly, disabled, recently had surgery, have a respiratory condition or viral infection, or have a compromised immune system.
- Viral pneumonia. This kind accounts for around one-third of all occurrences of pneumonia and is brought on by a variety of viruses, including the flu (influenza). If you have viral pneumonia, you can be more susceptible to developing bacterial pneumonia.
- Mycoplasma pneumonia. This form of pneumonia, which is referred to as atypical pneumonia, is characterized by symptoms and clinical manifestations that are slightly distinct from those of conventional pneumonia. Mycoplasma pneumonia is the bacteria that causes it. It typically results in a broad, moderate pneumonia that affects people of all ages.
- Other pneumonias. Other, less frequent pneumonias may be brought on by other organisms, such fungus.

Another crucial factor is where individuals are when they contract pneumonia. This is due to the fact that different varieties of bacteria exist in different environments. In comparison to organisms found in other contexts, those in certain environments, like hospitals, are usually more harmful and antibiotic-resistant. In some situations, people are also more likely to have conditions that increase their risk of developing pneumonia.

Individuals residing in the community can contract community-acquired pneumonia.

Pneumonia that has been contracted at a hospital is known as "hospital-acquired pneumonia."

Health care-associated pneumonia refers to an illness contracted outside of a hospital environment, such as a nursing home or a dialysis facility. It is classified as a subgroup of community-acquired pneumonia because these patients are more likely to have pneumonia caused by the same organisms that infect other people in the community.

3.1.3 Risk Factors for Pneumonia

Pneumonia may strike anybody at any time. But those who smoke, are older than 65, have certain medical issues, are younger than 2 years old, or are older adults have a higher chance of getting pneumonia.

Pneumonia can also occur as a consequence of trauma, particularly a chest injury, or after surgery, particularly abdominal surgery, as the discomfort from these diseases prevents patients from inhaling deeply and from coughing. Microorganisms are more likely to persist in the lungs and lead to illness if patients do not breathe deeply and cough. Additionally, persons who are bedridden, paralyzed, asleep, or disabled also are unable to breathe deeply and cough. These folks are also highly susceptible to pneumonia.

The presence of pneumonia in a healthy or immune-compromised individual is another crucial distinction. An individual with a compromised immune system is far more prone to get pneumonia, including pneumonia brought on by uncommon bacteria, viruses, fungi, or parasites. Moreover, a person with a compromised immune system would not react to treatment as effectively as someone with a robust immune system. A person's immune system may be compromised if they:

- Use certain medications
- Suffer from certain illnesses, such as cancer or the acquired immunodeficiency syndrome (AIDS)
- Have an underdeveloped immune system, as do newborns and young children.
- Have a severely weakened immune system as a result of sickness
- Alcoholism, smoking, diabetes, heart failure, being older than 65 years, and chronic obstructive pulmonary disease are some illnesses that predispose people to pneumonia because they might impair the immune system or the lungs' defence systems.

3.1.4 Complications of Pneumonia

Potential complications include

- Low concentrations of oxygen in the blood
- Critically low blood pressure levels
- Empyema or lung abscess
- Serious lung damage
- Breathlessness

The pneumonia-causing bacteria may enter the circulation, or the body may overreact to the infection, leading to a fall in blood pressure which can be fatal. Such a condition is known as sepsis.

Some pneumonias can cause an empyema or a lung abscess, which is a pus-filled pocket of tissue. Abscesses are developed when a tiny portion of the lung dies and a mass of pus accumulates in its stead. Whereas, an empyema is a buildup of pus in the area between the lung and the chest.

Acute respiratory distress syndrome (ARDS) can appear as a result of a severe lung damage, brought on by a bad infection or excessive inflammation brought on by the infection. Shortness of breath brought on by ARDS frequently involves shallow, fast breathing. People with ARDS typically need prolonged mechanical ventilation support for their breathing.

3.2 Pneumonia Dataset

Chest X-ray images (anterior-posterior) were selected from retrospective cohorts of pediatric patients of 1–5 years old from Guangzhou Women and Children's Medical Center, Guangzhou [7]. All chest X-ray imaging was performed as part of patients' routine clinical care.

The dataset was organized into 3 folders (train, test, val) with a total of 5863 X-ray images (JPEG) and 2 categories (pneumonia/normal) [7].

For the analysis of chest x-ray images, all chest radiographs were initially screened for quality control by removing all low quality or unreadable scans. The diagnoses for the images were then graded by two expert physicians before being cleared for training the AI system. In order to account for any grading errors, the evaluation set was also checked by a third expert.

3.3 Classifying Pneumonia

CNNs are deep neural networks, characterised by their high learning efficiency. CNNs have a wide variety of applications in the medical field such as disease analysis, image reading, patient classification, disease prediction and so on [12]. CNNs were used to aid the diagnosis of thoracic Computerised Tomography (CT) scans, during the outbreak of the novel acute infectious disease of COVID-19. CT image data of patients diagnosed with COVID-19 and those diagnosed with typical pneumonia were used to train a CNN model, achieving an area under the curve of up to 0.93 which represents the predictive power of this methodology. Using a CNN, The diagnosis time for a single case was determined to be 10 s [10]. Using conventional clinical indicators, other researchers such as Feng, used logistic regression to screen and sort a series of specific physiological indicators by importance. By observing the history of COVID-19 exposure during the early stage of the epidemic, a Lasso recursive machine learning algorithm was then established to be used as an auxiliary model for early diagnosis of suspected cases without the need for CT examination[2]. For predicting patient complications, Jiang et al. designed a model to predict ARDS in COVID-19 patients by using the data on confirmed cases with positive COVID-19 NUCLEIC acid tests for a throat swab. In addition, in data pre-treatment, 11 feature sets were determined as significant by the filtering method and used in model training, achieving good performance[3].

Here we will illustrate how the CNN model can be used to detect and classify pneumonia in CT scans of patient lungs. The images collected will go through a series of pre-processing. Model iteration and compilation will be carried out, and the accuracy of the model will be evaluated on the test set afterwards [6].

3.3.1 Methodology

Convolutional neural networks (CNNs) were inspired by biological processes, in that the connectivity pattern between neurons resembles the organization of the animal visual cortex. CNNs were first founded by Hubel and Wiesel and use relatively little pre-processing compared to other image classification algorithms. One reason is that the CNN network learns to optimize the weights of its filters (or kernels) through automated learning, whereas in traditional algorithms these filters are hand-engineered. This independence from prior knowledge and human intervention in feature extraction is a major advantage. The algorithm structure we used to solve this problem is as described below in Fig. 3.1.

Data Pre-processing

Initially, data processing is necessary and important. We used the functions of the opencv module to read the pictures in grayscale. We then reshaped the size of the pictures to a resolution of about 150 × 150. In this way, we could load, relatively easily, the pictures to the train matrix, test matrix and validation matrix. We also

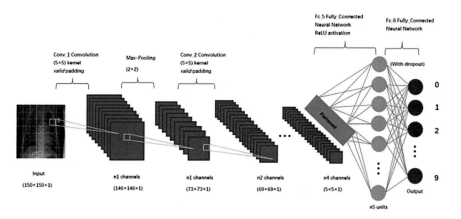

Fig. 3.1 The structure of the neural network

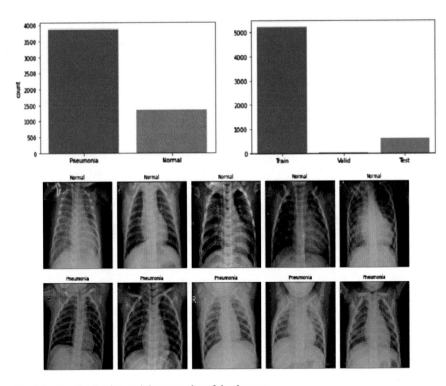

Fig. 3.2   The distribution and the examples of the data set

loaded the labels for the images simultaneously. To begin with, we needed to check the samples of the training set. Statistically, the distribution of the training set and the quantity of different values are as follows (Fig. 3.2).

We then used the function ImageDataGenerator, which is a useful tool to flip and shift the images randomly, so that we could get a more diverse training set. Though the whole process discussed above, we began to fit the training set into the convolution and pooling layers. The description of the convolution and pooling layers as follows. There have been many successful classifications which used CNNs[1]. In past research, Alexnet[11] and Resnet[13] achieved excellent performance in the classification of images. Compared to VGG16, Alexnet has fewer parameters to train, which means that it is easier for computers to calculate. Therefore, we integrated some characteristics of Alexnet in constructing our own network. However, due to the relatively small number of layers, we did not opt to add the residual as they did. We also aimed to design a relatively simple neural network to achieve the classification due to the potential gradient explosion. potential gradient explosion.

Convolution and Pooling Layers

The Convoluted Neural Network Algorithm is demonstrated as in Fig. 3.3.

In the first convolutional layer, the result equals the sum of the Hadamard product of the original image and the 5×5 filter. So the 150×150 image resulted in a 146×146 output, as in Fig. 3.4.

The pooling layer outputs the maximum value of each 2×2 matrix. The 146×146 image from the previous layer is used as input and the output shape is 73×73, as in Fig. 3.5.

For the first convolution layer, the parameters of this layer are as follows:

1. The number of filters is 16.
2. Convolution kernel size is 5×5.
3. Strider defaults to 1.
4. Padding defaults to valid, which means the boundary is not processed.
5. The size of the input shape is 150×150.
6. ReLU is used as the activation function.

The size of the output shape is 146×146. Then, in the first pooling layer, the parameters of this layer are as follows:

Fig. 3.3 The demonstration of the algorithm

Convoluted Neural Network Algorithm

Given:

training data: $(P_1, P_2, P_3, \cdots P_n)$, $P_i \in P$, the array of pictures(having been prepossessed); Epochs; $X \in P$, $X \in [-1, 1]$; training labels;

(Addition: P is a three-dimensional matrix correlated with RGB. Every single elements X of the matrix is a normalization factor).

Use AlexNet as the network structure. Set up and compile the convoluted neuron network(Fig.1). Initialize weights(W) of every cells.

For i in range Epochs:

For j in range P:

1. Get one sample P_j from P as the input of the neural network.
2. Through front propagation method(including the convolution, max-pooling, full connected, etc), get the output of the network.
3. Compare the output and the label, get the difference δ of it.
4. Use δ to do back propagation to update W which are needed to change.
5. Get the neural network with new W.
6. Use the new network to continue propagation.

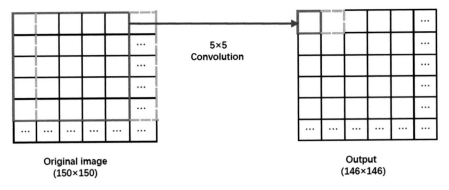

Fig. 3.4   The calculation of the first layer

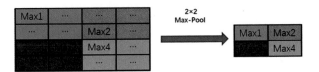

Fig. 3.5   The calculation of the max-pooling layer

1. Pool size is 2 × 2
2. Striders equal to 2.

The output shape is 73 × 73, and the filters are set as 32, 64 and 128 matrices, constructing another 6 layers (3 convolution layers and 3 pooling layers). After that the output shape becomes 5 × 5. Flatten and Fully Connected layers:

1. The Flatten function is used in the flatten layer.

    In the fully connected layer:

1. The number of units is 1024.
2. The activation function is ReLU.

Additionally, in the second layer, the number of units are changed to 256. While in the third layer, the number of units changed to 1 and the activation function to sigmoid. The whole structure is displayed as in Fig. 3.6.

3.3.2   Model Compilation

In this section, we outline the effect and the actual situation of model iteration. The model performed front propagation with different run times. We also recorded the actual accuracy of the model. In order to avoid overfitting or underfitting, we controlled the amount of epochs and digitally retained the clarity of the pictures,

Layer (type)	Output Shape	Param #
conv2d (Conv2D)	(None, 146,146,16)	416
max_pooling2d (Maxpooling2D)	(None, 73, 73, 16)	0
dropout (Dropout)	(None, 73, 73, 16)	0
conv2d_1 (Conv2D)	(None, 69, 69, 32)	12832
max_pooling2d_1 (MaxPooling2	(None, 34, 34, 32)	0
dropout-1 (Dropout)	(None, 34, 34, 32)	0
conv2d_2 (Conv2D)	(None, 30, 30, 64)	51264
max_pooling2d_2 (MaxPooling2	(None, 15, 15, 64)	0
dropout_2 (Dropout)	(None, 15, 15, 64)	0
conv2d_3 (Conv2D)	(None, 11, 11, 128)	204928
max_pooling2d_3 (MaxPooling2	(None, 5, 5, 128)	0
dropout_3 (Dropout)	(None, 5, 5, 128)	0
flatten (Flatten)	(None, 3200)	0
dense (Dense)	(None, 1024)	3277824
dropout_4 (Dropout)	(None, 1024)	0
dense_1 (Dense)	(None, 256)	262400
dropout_5 (Dropout)	(None, 256)	0
dense_2 (Dense)	(None, 1)	257

Total params: 3,809,921
Trainable params: 3,809,921
Non-trainable params: 0

Fig. 3.6 The structure of the first neural network

so that we can get enough information from the training data. There are different situations, connected with different iterative times, as follows. In addition, in an additional attempt to avoid overfitting learning, we partitioned some samples from the training dataset in advance as validation data. By observing the accuracy of the model on the validation dataset, we had a clear reference parameter to avoid overfitting.

Optimizer

We adopt the RMSprop optimizer to update the learning rate. When it comes to optimizers, AdaGrad is the most famous optimizer in machine learning. Notably, it updates the learning rate based on momentum. In comparison, RMSprop updates the learning rate through a more variable method. According to the RMSprop algorithm, taking y = kx + b as an example, it is assumed that the vertical axis represents parameter b and the horizontal axis represents parameter k. Since the value of k is greater than b, the contour of the whole gradient is elliptical. It can be seen that the closer points are to the lowest point (valley bottom), the greater the difference between the horizontal axis and the vertical axis of the ellipse, which corresponds to the valley terrain.

The gradient direction of each position is perpendicular to the contour line. Then, near the valley, although the horizontal axis is advancing, the swing amplitude of the vertical axis is also increasing, which is a phenomenon termed valley oscillation. If the random gradient drops too rapidly, it is likely to oscillate up and down continuously and not converge near the optimal value. Therefore, we slowed down adjustment in the direction of parameter b (vertical axis) and sped up adjustment in the direction of parameter k (horizontal axis). Meanwhile, we normalize the parameters, including k and b, so that we can change the elliptical graph into a circle graph, which is more convenient to update. In a word, RMSprop has the special ability to perform self-adaptive adjustment, compared to other kinds of optimizer. Nevertheless, this optimizer has some disadvantages which will be discussed in the section on model improvement. The optimizer progresses as in Fig. 3.7. And the optimizer progresses as in Fig. 3.7.

Loss

We adopt the binary cross entropy as the loss function. The binary cross entropy is one of the most popular loss functions in the machine learning. The calculation formula is as follows:

$$Loss = -\frac{1}{N} \sum_{i=1}^{N} y_i * log(p(y_i)) + (1 - y_i) * log(1 - p(y_i))$$

y is the binary label 0 or 1, and P(y) is the probability that the output belongs to the Y label. As a loss function, binary cross entropy is used to judge the quality of the prediction results of a binary classification model. Generally speaking, for the case where label y is 1, as the predicted value p(y) approaches 1, the value of the loss function should approach 0. On the contrary, if the predicted value p(y) approaches 0 at this time, the value of the loss function should be very large, which is very consistent with the nature of the log function.

RMSprop optimizer algorithm

1. Calculate the gratitude of every parameters:

$$dw_i = \frac{\partial L(w)}{\partial w_i}$$

2. Calculate the update amount:

$$s \times dw_i = \beta \times S \times dw_i + (1 - \beta) \times dw_i^2$$

(Notes: dw_i^2 equals the square of dw_i)

3. Update the parameters:

$$w_i = w_i - \eta \frac{dw_i}{\sigma + \sqrt{Sdw_i}}$$

(Notes: σ is a small positive numbers in case $\sqrt{Sdw_i} = 0$)

Fig. 3.7 The process of the RMSprop optimizer algorithm

Compilation

After choosing the optimizer and the method of calculating the loss, we inputted our samples into the model and recorded the fitting process. We used the validation datasets to monitor the performance. In the process of compilation, we found the loss and the accuracy on the training datasets to change constantly. However, through analysis of the record, we found that the model after 30 epochs was more likely to have ideal performance. When the epochs exceed 30, accuracy did not obviously rise and sometimes went down because of possible overfitting.

3.3.3 Model Evaluation

Although deep learning and neural networks are widely used in the field of medical imaging and have significant effects, it is very important to evaluate a trained model. Moreover, it is necessary to ensure accuracy of recognition as much as possible in the field of health. Therefore, in order to analyze the usability of the model, we have adopted a variety of methods and analyzed the model from different dimensions.

Accuracy

First, we analyzed the accuracy of the model. Accuracy represents the rate of correct predictions, and the definition of accuracy is as follows:

$$Accuracy = \frac{TP + TN}{P + N}$$

After evaluating:The accuracy of the model is approximately 91.186 %.

In addition, we analyzed the accuracy of the model across different epochs again. After comparison, we find that when the epoch is 30, the accuracy and loss of the test set of the model are the smallest, as in Fig. 3.8.

Even though the accuracy held up well, it was not convincing due to the problem of an uneven sample data. If the samples in the training set are not balanced, the accuracy may be very high and it does not mean that the classifier is effective. This will cause a lot of trouble to the doctor using the classifier.

LogLoss

In order to evaluate the loss of the model more accurately. We used LogLoss to estimate the degree of inconsistency between the model's predicted value f(x) and the true value Y.

After evaluating: Loss of the model is −0.4290.

Logloss measures the difference between the actual probability distribution and the probability distribution estimated by the model. Here, lower is better. In addition, LogLoss is sensitive to the estimated probability, which means that even if the positive and negative samples of the training set are not balanced, it retains much of its effectiveness. For example, though the data set has many negative samples and few positive samples, we hope to be able to identify more positive samples while controlling for false positives. However, if no optimization is made to the model, LogLoss tends to be biased towards the negative sample. In such situations, the LogLoss may be very low, but the recognition effect of the model for identifying positive samples would not be ideal in live application.

Precision and Recall

We also used Precision and Recall to further evaluate the effect of the model. Precision refers to the percentage of samples judged as "true" by the system that were actually true. The definition of Precision is as follows:

$$Precision = \frac{TP}{TP + FP}$$

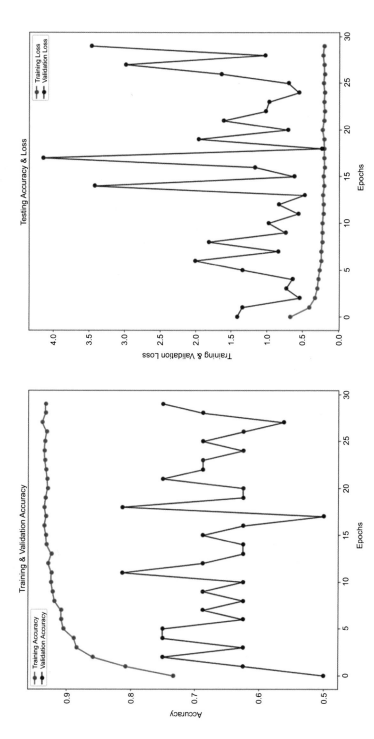

Fig. 3.8 The variation curve of accuracy and loss

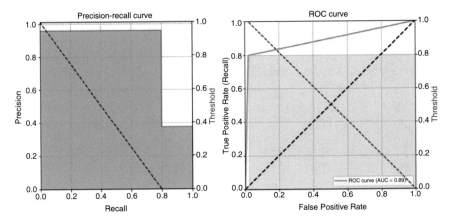

Fig. 3.9 The precision-recall curve and ROC curve

Recall refers to the proportion of samples correctly judged as "true" to all samples correctly judged by the model. The definition of Recall is as follows:

$$Recall = \frac{TP}{TP + TN}$$

After evaluating:

- Precision of the model is approximately 0.9590
- Recall of the model is approximately 0.7991

In the context of pneumonia detection, precision represents the proportion of patients who have not been misdiagnosed, while recall represents the diagnosis rate of patients with pneumonia. In this application, precision and recall are both important, because it is necessary to both avoid misdiagnosing healthy people as pneumonia patients, and to also screen out pneumonia patients from the crowd as much as possible to avoid group infections. Therefore, the model must comprehensively consider precision and recall. The ROC curves and PR curves are shown as in Fig. 3.9.

F1 Score

By using F1-Score, both precision and recall can be simultaneously used to evaluate the misdiagnosis rate and screening rate of the model. After evaluation, the F1 of the model is approximately 0.8718.The confusion matrix is displayed as in Fig. 3.10.

Analysis of the confusion matrix suggests that there are a large quantity of images which are wrongly classified. There are also some other problems, which will be discussed in model improvement, with the model. Therefore, a new structure was decided on to solve the problem.

	Predicted Normal	Predicted Pneumonia
Actual Normal	382	8
Actual Pneumonia	47	187

Fig. 3.10 The confusion matrix of the first model

3.3.4 Model Improvement

Model evaluation revealed that after 30 epochs, the accuracy of the model could reach over 91%, which seemed good enough for auxiliary diagnosis. However, we noticed, during the experiment, that sometimes, the accuracy oscillated around a constant, like around 74%, and did not increase as the number of iterations increased. Based on our analysis, we concluded that this phenomenon was caused by the relatively large learning rate that can not decline in time, which results in the failure of the gradient descent algorithm. One solution would be to constantly adjust the random seed and learning rate to try to tackle it, another would be to construct a new model. However, considering the low performance on other tests, we came up with a new network to solve the problem. In the new network, we reduced the size of the convolution kernels and also changed the size of the pictures in order to ensure that the network could get more information per image. Undoubtedly, the larger size of the images, the more information the model could analyze. However, we also needed to consider the time cost, which increases with the square of the picture size. After a few attempts, we found that 256×256 images were more likely to offer a good balance between performance and run time.

Meanwhile, we also compare several optimizers to figure the most appropriate optimizer for the model, and through experiments, we find the Adam optimizer more efficient[8], solving the problem of oscillating accuracy and increasing general accuracy[5]. According to several past dissertations, the Adam optimizer always has better performance than RMSprop. The main difference between two optimizers is that the Adam has the ability to do the deviation correction, which ensures that it can tackle large quantities of samples, and is particularly effective for images with sparse gradients.

The methods of calculating effectiveness have been discussed above comprehensively and will not be further tackled. The structure of the new network is in Fig. 3.11.

In terms of structure, the total parameters are fewer than the former model. Due to the more detailed information from the images, the time cost is more than the former network per epoch, at about 56 s using the RTX 2060. This is about five times longer than the former network per epoch. But the advantage is that every layer will have much more information to utilize, which means that the neural network will be less likely to be overfitted. During the compilation, we also performed thirty iterations and observed the performance. We found that the training accuracy was much better

Layer (type)	Output Shape	Param #
conv2d (Conv2D)	(None, 254, 254, 32)	320
max_pooling2d (Maxpooling2D)	(None, 127, 127, 32)	0
dropout (Dropout)	(None, 127, 127, 32)	0
conv2d_1 (Conv2D)	(None, 125, 125, 32)	9248
max_pooling2d_1 (MaxPooling2	(None, 62, 62, 32)	0
dropout-1 (Dropout)	(None, 62, 62, 32)	0
conv2d_2 (Conv2D)	(None, 60, 60, 64)	18496
max_pooling2d_2 (MaxPooling2	(None, 30, 30, 64)	0
dropout_2 (Dropout)	(None, 30, 30, 64)	0
conv2d_3 (Conv2D)	(None, 28, 28, 64)	36928
max_pooling2d_3 (MaxPooling2	(None, 14, 14, 64)	0
dropout_3 (Dropout)	(None, 14, 14, 64)	0
flatten (Flatten)	(None, 12544)	0
dense (Dense)	(None, 256)	3211520
dropout_4 (Dropout)	(None, 256)	0
dense_1 (Dense)	(None, 1)	257

```
Total params: 3,276,769
Trainable params: 3,276,769
Non-trainable params: 0
```

Fig. 3.11 The structure of the new neural network

than the former model, and the test accuracy a little higher than the former model. The changes in the loss and the accuracy are demonstrated in Fig. 3.12.

The confusion matrix is recorded as in Fig. 3.13.

More specifically, the training accuracy for classifying pneumonia is about 95.260%, while the test accuracy of classifying is about 91.987%. Meanwhile, the other parameters used to evaluate the model are as follows (Fig. 3.14): Precision of the model is approximately 0.8290 Recall of the model is approximately 0.9820 F1 of the model is approximately 0.8990

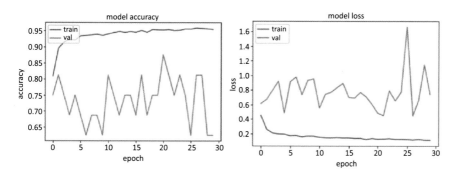

Fig. 3.12 Model accuracy and model loss

	Predicted Normal	Predicted Pneumonia
Actual Normal	191	43
Actual Pneumonia	7	383

Fig. 3.13 The confusion matrix of the new model

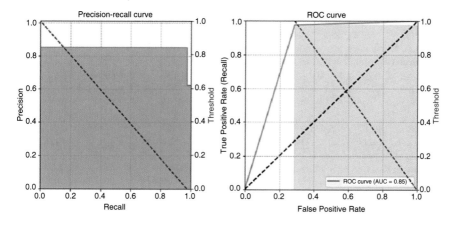

Fig. 3.14 ROC curve and precision-recall curve

Actually, from observation, the outcome implies that more detailed images may cause a reduction in precision, but they can increase the training accuracy and the test accuracy as well as the balance between precision and recall—the F1. Additionally, we can use several neural networks to help us to get a comprehensive result, which may be a more efficient way in the prediction.

3.3.5   Conclusion

In conclusion, we have shown how to develop a pneumonia classification algorithm using X-ray images and CNNs. We found the best performing model to be trained for 30 epochs. The accuracy of this model was 91.186%, the loss of the model is 0.4290, the precision of the model is 0.9590, and the recall of the model is 0.7991. We then further optimized the model by changed the convolution kernels and replaced the Adam optimizer with the RMSprop optimizer. According to the new results, the model's accuracy in classifying pneumonia is about 91.987%, and the precision of the model is 0.8290 while the recall of the model is 0.9820, and the F1 of the model is 0.8990.

References

1. Das, P. K., & Meher, S. (2021). An efficient deep convolutional neural network based detection and classification of acute lymphoblastic leukemia. *Expert Systems with Applications, 183*, 115311.
2. Feng, C., Wang, L., Chen, X., Zhai, Y., Zhu, F., Chen, H., Wang, Y., Su, X., Huang, S., Tian, L., Zhu, W., Sun, W., Zhang, L., Han, Q., Zhang, J., Pan, F., Chen, L., Zhu, Z., Xiao, H., . . . Li, T. (2021). A novel triage tool of artificial intelligence-assisted diagnosis aid system for suspected covid-19 pneumonia in fever clinics. *medRxiv*.
3. Jiang, X., Coffee, M., Bari, A., Wang, J., Jiang, X., Huang, J., Shi, J., Dai, J., Cai, J., Zhang, T., Wu, Z., He, G., & Huang, Y. (2020). Towards an artificial intelligence framework for data-driven prediction of coronavirus clinical severity. *Computers, Materials & Continua, 63*(1), 537–551.
4. John Hopkins Medicine. Pneumonia.
5. Liu, X. (2021). Research on the forecast of coal price based on LSTM with improved Adam optimizer. *Journal of Physics: Conference Series, 1941*(1), 012069.
6. Liu, J., Zhao, W., Li, Z., Song, Z., & Teoh, T. T. (2022). Pneumonia image classification method based on improved convolutional neural network. In *2022 IEEE international conference on electrical engineering, big data and algorithms (EEBDA)*.
7. Mooney, P. (2018). Chest x-ray images (pneumonia).
8. Ramalingam, V. V., & Ragavendran, R. (2020). Prediction of liver disease using artificial neural network with Adam optimizer. *Journal of Critical Reviews, 7*(17), 1287–1292.
9. Sethi, S. (2022). Overview of pneumonia - lung and airway disorders.
10. Wang, S., Kang, B., Ma, J., Zeng, X., Xiao, M., Guo, J., Cai, M., Yang, J., Li, Y., Meng, X., & Xu, B. (2020). A deep learning algorithm using ct images to screen for corona virus disease (covid-19). *medRxiv*.
11. Xiao, X., Yang, H., Yi, W., Wan, Y., Huang, Q., & Lou, J. (2021). Application of improved alexnet model in rice pest image recognition. *Science Technology and Engineering, 21*(22), 9447–9454.
12. Zhang, C. (2021). Application of ai technology in diagnosis and treatment of covid-19. *Chinese Journal of Medical Instrumentation, 45*(04), 372–375.
13. Zhao, C. (2021). Application of image classification based on resnet18 in crop pest diagnosis. *Agriculture and Technology, 41*(19), 10–13.

Chapter 4
CNN for White Blood Cell Classification

4.1 Introduction to White Blood Cells

As the blood circulates through the body, blood cells, which are present in the blood, can move about the body. Red blood cells, white blood cells, and platelets make up the majority of blood cells in humans. The primary job of red blood cells is to carry oxygen. White blood cells primarily provide an immunological function. When germs infiltrate the body, white blood cells can penetrate the capillary wall, focus on the invasion site, encircle the bacteria, and swallow them. In the process of hemostasis, the process to stop bleeding, platelets are crucial.

Red blood cells, white blood cells, and platelets together make up around 45% of the blood volume. Under normal conditions, blood cells and platelets have a certain morphological form and a comparatively constant quantity. Therefore, numerous illnesses may be discovered by analyzing the form, quantity, and other characteristics of many kinds of blood cells.

When you have too many or too few white blood cells, you might have white blood cell diseases [1]. White blood cells, are one of the four different kinds of blood cells. They are made in the bone marrow and are crucial to the functioning of your immune system. ·

A test known as a white blood cell (WBC) count allows doctors to monitor these cells. White blood cell counts that are excessively high often indicate that your immune system is actively battling an infection or illness. When they are abnormally low, your immune system may have been compromised by an illness, autoimmune disorder, or other condition.

A white blood cell count can frequently be the first indication of an illness and can provide some insight as to the type of disease you may have, even though it cannot be used to diagnose any medical condition.

Additionally, there are five main categories of white blood cells, each of which has a particular purpose: Basophils, Eosinophils, Lymphocytes, Neutrophils, and Monocytes

T. T. Teoh, *Convolutional Neural Networks for Medical Applications*, SpringerBriefs in Computer Science, https://doi.org/10.1007/978-981-19-8814-1_4

There are illnesses that solely affect a single variety of white blood cell, whereas others can impact a wide variety. For example, lymphocytic leukocytosis is a condition that only affects lymphocytes, whereas neutrophilic leukocytosis is a condition that only affects neutrophils. Doctors can determine the sort of disease a patient has based on the cells that are impacted.

4.2   White Blood Cells Dataset

This dataset contains 12,500 augmented images of blood cells with accompanying cell type labels [5]. There are approximately 3000 images for each of 4 different cell types. The cell types are Eosinophil, Lymphocyte, Monocyte, and Neutrophil.

4.2.1   Eosinophil

White blood cells known as eosinophils are crucial to the body's response to allergic responses, asthma attacks, and parasitic infections [7]. These cells not only play a part in the inflammation that results from allergic illnesses, but they also play a part in the defense response against certain parasites.

Eosinophils induce inflammation in some organs, resulting in symptoms.

Eosinophils typically make up less than 7% of the white blood cells in circulation (between 100 and 500 per microliter of blood [0.1 and 0.5×109 per liter]).

Low Eosinophil Count

Eosinopenia, which refers to a low concentration of eosinophils in the blood, can be brought on by Cushing syndrome, bloodstream infections (sepsis), and corticosteroid therapy. However, a low eosinophil count normally doesn't create issues since other components of our immune system can make up for it.

A low amount of eosinophils is frequently discovered by coincidence when a full blood count is performed for a separate reason.

Treatment of the underlying cause restores the usual quantity of eosinophils.

High Eosinophil Count

The most frequent reasons of a high eosinophil count (also known as hypereosinophilia or eosinophilia) include

- Allergies
- Parasite infections
- Some types of cancer

Eosinophil counts are frequently raised by allergic conditions, sensitivity to certain medicines, asthma, allergic rhinitis, and atopic dermatitis. Many parasites can induce eosinophilia, especially those which penetrate tissue. Hodgkin lymphoma, leukemia, and certain myeloproliferative neoplasms are cancers that can result in eosinophilia.

People often have no symptoms if the blood eosinophil count is just slightly higher than normal. High blood eosinophil count is only identified after a full blood count is performed for some other reason. However, occasionally when the eosinophil count is extremely high, the increased eosinophil count damages organs and inflames tissues. Although any organ can be harmed, the heart, lungs, skin, and nervous system are most frequently impacted.

Symptoms depend on which organ is hurt. When a person's skin is impacted, for instance, they may develop a rash; when their lungs are affected, they may experience wheezing and shortness of breath; when their heart is affected, they may experience shortness of breath and exhaustion (symptoms of heart failure); and when their esophagus or stomach is affected, they may have discomfort in their throat and stomach. As a result, eosinophilic diseases are classified according to the region where eosinophil levels are elevated: As a result, eosinophilic diseases are classified according to the region where eosinophil levels are elevated.

In most cases, a person's symptoms are initially evaluated and treated for more widespread causes. For instance, even if no infection is discovered, they might still undergo testing for it and even receive antibiotics. When patients continue to experience symptoms while receiving therapy, doctors frequently take a tissue sample for analysis (biopsy), which reveals the presence of eosinophils in the damaged organ.

Oral corticosteroids are often used in the treatment of these disorders.

4.2.2 Lymphocyte

White blood cells known as lymphocytes have a variety of functions in the immune system, including defense against bacteria, viruses, fungi, and parasites [9]. 20–40% of the white blood cells in the circulation are typically lymphocytes. In adults, the lymphocyte count typically exceeds 1500 cells per microliter of blood (1.5×10^9 cells per liter), whereas in children, it typically exceeds 3000 cells per microliter of blood (3×10^9 cells per liter). A decrease in the number of lymphocytes may not result in a significant fall in the overall number of white blood cells.

Three different kinds of lymphocytes exist:

1. B lymphocytes (B cells)
2. T lymphocytes (T cells)
3. Natural killer cells (NK cells)

The immune system relies on all three kinds of lymphocytes in crucial ways. An Infections or cancer could cause an increase in any of the three types. In certain situations, however, the count of just one kind of lymphocyte is elevated. The number of plasma cells, which make antibodies, might drop if there are not enough B cells. Bacterial infections would also rise as antibody production declines.

Too few T cells or NK cells make it difficult for some illnesses to be controlled, including parasitic, fungal, and viral infections. Serious lymphocyte shortages can lead to uncontrolled infections that can be deadly.

Low Lymphocyte Count

The quantity of lymphocytes in the blood can be decreased by a number of diseases and circumstances, including infection with viruses such the influenza virus, SARS-CoV-2, and the AIDS-causing human immunodeficiency virus (HIV) [9]. This disease is called Lymphocytopenia, also otherwise known as lymphopenia.

Lymphocyte count might drop during:

- A few viral illnesses (such as influenza, hepatitis, and COVID-19)
- Fasting
- Extreme physical stress
- Corticosteroid use (such as prednisone)
- Cancer treatment with chemotherapy and/or radiation

Doctors often do a blood test for the presence of the human immunodeficiency virus (HIV) and other infections when the number of lymphocytes is significantly decreased. In certain cases, a sample of bone marrow is also collected for microscopic analysis (bone marrow examination).

It is also possible to identify the types of particular lymphocyte subtypes in the blood (T cells, B cells, and NK cells). A reduction in specific kinds of lymphocytes may assist doctors in diagnosing certain diseases, such as AIDS or genetic immunodeficiency disorders.

High Lymphocyte Count

Lymphocytosis is the condition where there is an above average count of Lymphocytes in the body. The most prevalent reason for an increase in lymphocytes is viral infection (such as mononucleosis) [8]. The number may also rise as a result of some bacterial illnesses, such TB. Acute or chronic lymphocytic leukemia, lymphomas, and other cancers may cause a rise in lymphocytes in the body, in part by releasing immature lymphocytes (lymphoblasts) or lymphoma cells into the bloodstream. The quantity of lymphocytes in the circulation may also rise as a result of Graves disease and Crohn's disease.

Typically, there are no symptoms associated with an increase in lymphocytes. However, the increase in lymphocytes may result in fever, night sweats, and weight loss in persons with lymphoma and certain leukemias [8]. Additionally, rather than being directly related to the rise in lymphocytes, symptoms may arise from the infection or other condition that has generated them.

4.2.3   Monocyte

Monocytes are a kind of white blood cell that help other white blood cells remove dead or damaged tissues, eliminate cancer cells, and control immunity against foreign substances [10]. They also fight some diseases.

Monocytes are formed in the bone marrow and subsequently enter the bloodstream, where they account for around 1–10% of the circulating white blood cells (200–600 monocytes per microliter of blood [0.2–0.6 ×109 cells per liter]). After a few hours in the blood, monocytes move to tissues like the spleen, liver, lungs, and bone marrow, where they mature into macrophages.

The immune system's primary scavenger cells are macrophages. Certain genetic anomalies impair monocyte and macrophage activity and result in a buildup of fatty (lipid) waste inside the cells. The illnesses that develop as a result are known as lipid storage diseases (such as Gaucher disease and Niemann-Pick disease).

Monocyte counts, whether low or high, seldom result in symptoms. People, however, could exhibit signs of the disease which altered their monocyte count.

Low Monocyte Count

Infection in the bloodstream, chemotherapy, or a problem with the bone marrow can all result in monocytopenia, which would be a low level of monocytes in the blood [10].

High Monocyte Count

Chronic infections, autoimmune diseases, blood problems, and certain malignancies all result in an increase of monocytes in the blood (monocytosis) [10]. Infections, sarcoidosis, and Langerhans cell histiocytosis can all lead to an increase of macrophages in areas of the body other than the blood (including the lungs, skin, and other organs).

4.2.4   Neutrophil

White blood cells called neutrophils operate as the body's main line of defense against acute bacterial infections and some types of fungal infections [11]. About 45–75% of the white blood cells in the blood are typically neutrophils. Without the crucial defense that neutrophils offer, people struggle to control infections and run the danger of infection-related death.

About 1500 cells per microliter of blood, or 1.5×109 cells per liter, is the average lower limit of the neutrophil count. The danger of infection rises when the count falls below this mark.

Low Neutrophil Count

Neutropenia is characterized by an unusually low level of neutrophils, a particular type of white blood cell, in the blood [11].
The degree of neutropenia is categorized as:

- Mild: 1000–1500/mcL (1–1.5×109/L)
- Moderate: 500–1000/mcL (0.5–1×109/L)
- Severe: below 500/mcL (0.5×109/L)

The risk of infection significantly increases when the neutrophil count drops to less than 500 cells per microliter (severe neutropenia). Even the bacteria that would ordinarily exist in the mouth and intestines of a healthy person might potentially cause infections in such people.

Although there are several causes of neutropenia, there are mostly two types:

Neutrophils are depleted or destroyed quicker than bone marrow can replenish them. There is a decrease in the number of neutrophils produced in the bone marrow.

Many diseases cause neutrophils to be depleted or killed [11]. These conditions include a few bacterial infections, a few allergy conditions, and a few pharmacological therapies (such as drugs used to treat hyperthyroidism). People who have autoimmune diseases may produce antibodies that kill neutrophils and cause neutropenia. It is possible for individuals who have an enlarged spleen to have a low neutrophil count due to the fact that the bigger spleen captures and kills neutrophils

A decrease in neutrophil production in the bone marrow can be caused by cancer, influenza viruses, TB bacteria, myelofibrosis, or deficits of vitamin B12 or folate (folic acid). Neutropenia can also occur in patients who have undergone radiation therapy that affects the bone marrow.

Numerous medications, such as phenothiazine, sulfa medicines, many chemotherapy agents, as well as several toxins (benzene and insecticides), can also decrease the bone marrow's capacity to create neutrophils.

Aplastic anemia, a condition, also affects the bone marrow's ability to produce neutrophils (in which the bone marrow may shut down production of all blood cells).

Neutrophil counts can fall as a result of some uncommon genetic conditions. In cyclic neutropenia, neutrophil counts periodically fluctuate over the course of many weeks. Although infections are uncommon in chronic benign neutropenia, neutrophil counts are low, most likely because people manufacture just sufficient neutrophils in response to infection. People with severe congenital neutropenia, a series of diseases that prevent neutrophils from maturing, have severe infections as early as infancy.

High Neutrophil Count

An excessively high concentration of neutrophils in the blood is known as neutrophilic leukocytosis [12].

There are a variety of illnesses or ailments that might cause an increase in neutrophils, including:

- Infections
- Injuries
- Inflammatory disorders
- Certain drugs
- Certain leukemias

The body's typical reaction to an infection is the most likely explanation for an increase in neutrophils. In many cases, the body's increased production of neutrophils is an essential response as it works to repair or fight off an invading germ or foreign material. There may be an increase in neutrophils in the blood due to infections with bacteria, viruses, fungi, and parasites [12].

When someone has an injury, such as a hip fracture or burn, their neutrophil count may increase. Inflammatory illnesses, particularly autoimmune conditions like rheumatoid arthritis, can produce an increase in neutrophil quantity and activity. Some medications, such as corticosteroids, cause an increase in neutrophils in the blood. Myeloid leukemias can cause the blood to have more immature and mature neutrophils.

A high neutrophil count might not be symptomatic. However, the condition that is generating the elevated neutrophil count often has symptoms.

In exceedingly rare cases, excessively high numbers of immature neutrophils (more than 100,000 cells per microliter of blood [100×109 per liter]) can cause the blood to become overly thick, which can lead to difficulty breathing, stroke, and even death in patients who have leukemia. This situation is a medical emergency that necessitates hospitalization in order to administer intravenous fluids and medications to lower the white blood cell count (hydroxyurea and chemotherapeutic medicines). Sometimes, a procedure known as leukapheresis, which is a sort of therapy that filters the blood, is used to remove white blood cells from the blood.

4.3   Classifying White Blood Cells

The peripheral blood microscopy can well identify blood cell morphological characteristics and play an important role in the diagnosis and treatment of blood diseases such as lymphoma and leukemia. However, blood cell morphology analysis relies heavily on artificial microscopy, and there are inevitable errors and laborintensive status quo. Therefore, it is particularly important to develop a digital image analysis system that automatically classifies peripheral blood smears.

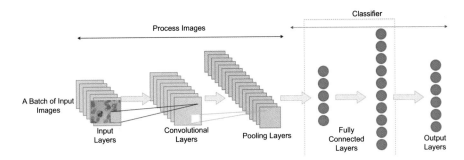

Fig. 4.1 A typical structure of CNN classifier

Automated methods through the use of Convolutional Neural Networks in Deep Learning, to count and classify blood cell subtypes, have important medical applications as it may indicate the presence of a White Blood Cell disease. We will develop a blood cell classification algorithm utilizing CNNs through practical optimization (Fig. 4.1).

4.3.1 EfficientNet

Model Structure (EfficientNet Model)

As shown in the Fig. 4.2, the structure of EfficientNet is quite complex: including a stem, 7 blocks and final layers. For each block, it can be reduced into 3 kinds of sub-block. And all the sub-blocks can be built by five kinds of module. After using EfficientNet model to get the feature of the images, a classifier with 2 fully-connected layers is connected (Fig. 4.3).

Advantage of EfficientNet Model

From the research in the past few years, we can see that to optimize the model, the scale of CNN is larger and larger to get a better performance. However, from [6], it states that the past model optimizations were focused on scaling only one dimension like resolution [13], depth [4] or width [3]. By scaling depth, richer and more complex features can be extracted from the images, while scaling width and resolution can capture more fine-granted features and increase accuracy. But when all these scaling performing singularly, there exists a bottleneck that the saturation appears quickly, which means that after scaling to some extent, further scaling didn't show apparent improvement. In other words, after saturation, even though the number of layers of the model is much higher than before, the accuracy of the model will not increase. To solve this problem, EfficientNet model scales the width, depth,

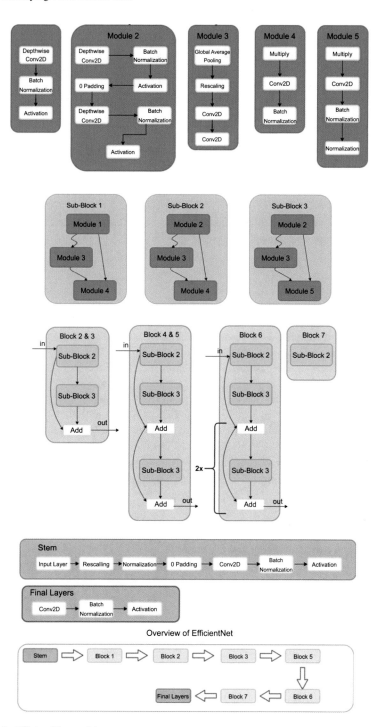

Fig. 4.2 EfficientNet model

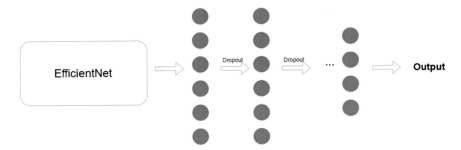

Fig. 4.3 Entire structure

and resolution uniformly to get a better performance and alleviates the bottleneck. The formulas are represented below:

$$d = \alpha^{\Phi}$$

$$w = \beta^{\Phi}$$

$$r = \gamma^{\Phi}$$

$$\alpha \cdot \beta^2 \cdot \gamma^2 \approx 2, \alpha \geq 1, \beta \geq 1, \gamma \geq 1$$

where d, w, r represent depth, width, resolution, and α, β, γ are three constants that can be calculated by grid search. Φ is a coefficient that determines the computation resource that can be used for scaling. More than that, the number of parameters of EfficientNet is much smaller, but the accuracy is much higher. So, it indicates that the speed of EfficientNet is higher without decreasing the accuracy. It's suitable for the situation in hospital: high accuracy and speed are needed at the same time.

4.3.2   Experimental Study

Preprocessing Data

Resize

The dataset we use contains 12,444 images of 4 kinds of white blood cells (as shown in Fig. 4.4): eosinophil, lymphocyte, monocyte, and neutrophil as the label of 1, 2, 3, 4 correspondingly. To cut down the data size that the model needs to process, all the images are resized to 80×60 before training. This step significantly decreases the time of training without losing high accuracy (Fig. 4.5).

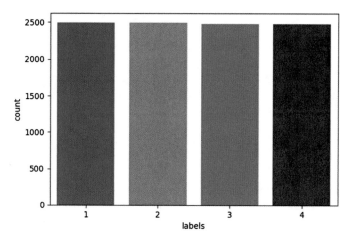

Fig. 4.4 The number of 4 kinds of white blood cells

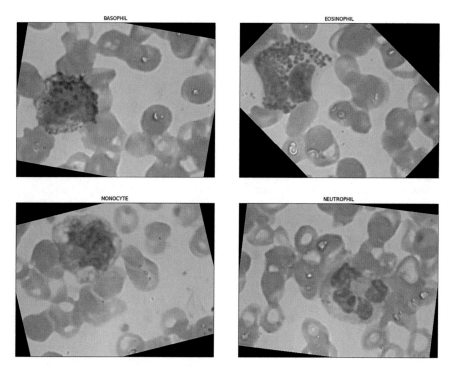

Fig. 4.5 Transformed images

Transform

Since the images used in the hospital can't be perfectly processed. Before putting into the model, all the images in the training set are randomly rotated in the range of 10° and randomly shifted by 10% compared to the original images. By this way, the generalization of the model can be improved [2] and make a better prediction even though the images are distorted.

Shuffle and Split

The dataset we get is organized in the order of classifications. The gradient descent method has its best performance when the instances are distributed uniformly and independently. So, it's necessary to randomly reorder the dataset. After that, the entire dataset is split into training set, validation set and test set for 80%, 5% 15% each.

Training Model

Pre-training

First of all, we set the training with the optimizer Adamax, which is stable and fast as we require. The learning rate was set as 0.01. Because of the classification was represented in numbers, the loss function we used was sparse categorical cross entropy. Then the EfficientNet model is loaded by TensorFlow. However, before the training began, we froze the layers in EfficientNet and pre-train the fully connected layers by 5 epochs. The reason was that the layers of loaded model have already learned some feature of images, and if we start with training the whole model, there is a possibility that the weights of the original model will be damaged. After pre-training, the EfficientNet layers were unfrozen and the learning rate was set to be 0.001 to avoid change the weights too much.

Adjust Learning Rate and Optimizer Dynamically and Early Stopping

Learning rate is a parameter that determines how much the parameters of model updated at each step. It's a very important parameter in the training process. If the training rate is too high, though the speed of training is fast at first, the loss will keep fluctuating or even keep increasing at the last few epochs. If the learning rate is too low, the model will be trained too slow and takes a lot of time for getting fully trained. During the training procedure, we recorded the best accuracy and loss at the end of each epoch. At first, we monitored the accuracy since the loss dropped quickly at the beginning. If the accuracy decreases than last epoch, the learning rate will decrease by the factor we set. Then after the accuracy met the threshold

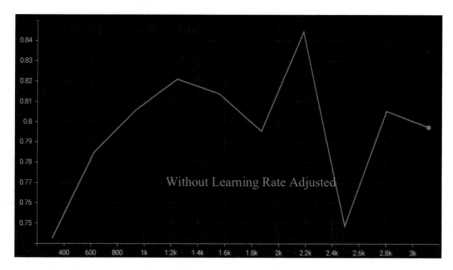

Fig. 4.6 Evaluation accuracy vs iterations

that we set, the validation loss was monitored. At the same time, the optimizer will be switch to stochastic gradient descent (SGD) with momentum 0.9. This is important, because in the field of computer vision, the optimizer of Adamax or some other adaptive optimizers tend to find a sharp minima, which is harmful for generalization. And SGD performs much better in this problem. However, at the beginning of training, Adamax optimizer was used due to its high speed, which helps increasing accuracy quickly. In this training set, it takes less than 2 min (2 epochs) to reach 97% accuracy in training set. When the validation loss increases, the learning rate will decrease similarly as the first stage (monitoring accuracy). If the performance does not increase for 5 epochs, the training will stop and the weight will be set as the same as that in the best epoch, which saves a lot of time and avoids training uselessly. Figure 4.6 compares the performance with and without adjusted learning rate.

Regularization

EfficientNet model is quite complicated that it has the risk of overfitting. So, the regularization is necessary. When the neural network is deeper, it's easier for the problem of vanishing gradient to happen. To alleviate this problem, batch normalization and skip connection were used. As for the fully-connected layer we use l1 regularization on bias and l2 regularization on weights. After one full-connected layer, a dropout layer with the rate of 0.45 was used.

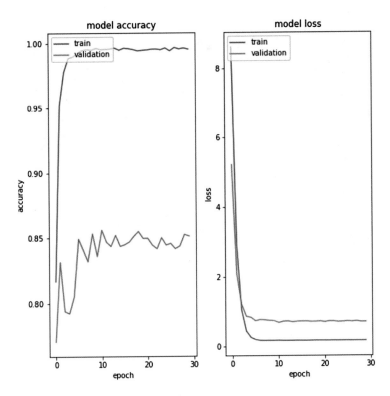

Fig. 4.7 Model accuracy vs model loss

Results and Evaluation

The procedure of training takes about 29 s per epoch (on a laptop with GPU RTX 3060), and within 5 epochs the accuracy of training set reaches 99%, which is fast enough for using practically. The test set was used to evaluate the trained model. Although the training accuracy reached more than 99%, it is still very important to evaluate the model. To quantize the usability of this model, we use precision, recall, F1 score and loss as indicators to evaluate it. Figures 4.7, 4.8 and 4.9 are the results.

$$Precision = \frac{TruePositive}{TruePositive + FalsePositive}$$

$$Recall = \frac{TruePositive}{TruePositive + FalseNegative}$$

$$F_1 = 2 \cdot \frac{Precision \cdot Recall}{Precision + Recall}$$

	precision	recall	f1-score	support
NEUTROPHIL	0.71	0.91	0.79	624
EOSINOPHIL	0.84	0.82	0.83	623
MONOCYTE	1.00	0.73	0.84	620
LYMPHOCYTE	1.00	1.00	1.00	620
accuracy			0.86	2487
macro avg	0.89	0.86	0.87	2487
weighted avg	0.89	0.86	0.87	2487

Fig. 4.8 The result of test set

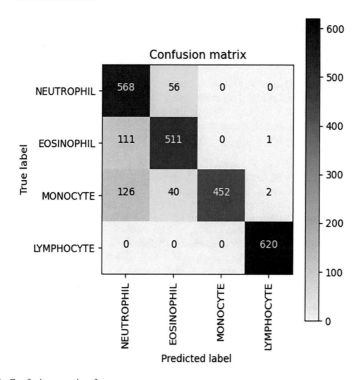

Fig. 4.9 Confusion matrix of test set

From Fig. 4.7, the learning curve of training set and validation set are becoming stable after 10th epoch, which means the model fits well. After evaluating, the loss of validation set is 0.69. As for the formulas above, True Positive means the prediction is correct. False Positive means that the model predict other class as this class, and False Negative means that predict this class as other class. The higher of F1 score, the better this model's prediction. The precision and recall are two contradictory quantities that if the precision is higher, the recall will be lower. And F1 score is a balance score of these two quantities. Only when both precision and recall are high and close to each other, the F1 score will be high. From Fig. 4.8, the F1 score of this model is 87%, which is competent to manage the task in hospital.

4.3.3   Conclusion

By using a CNN classifier based on EfficientNet model and making practical optimizations, the model is able to successfully identify different classes of white blood cells with a high speed and the accuracy of 90%. The accuracy reaches more than 90% in this dataset even with the interference of red blood cells.

References

1. Amber, Y. (2021). Overview of white blood cell disorders: Symptoms, diagnosis, treatment.
2. Das, P. K., & Meher, S. (2021). An efficient deep convolutional neural network based detection and classification of acute lymphoblastic leukemia. *Expert Systems with Applications, 183*, 115311.
3. Huang, G., Liu, Z., & Weinberger, K. Q. (2016). Densely connected convolutional networks. *CoRR*, abs/1608.06993.
4. Huang, G., Sun, Y., Liu, Z., Sedra, D., & Weinberger, K. Q. (2016). Deep networks with stochastic depth. In B. Leibe, J. Matas, N. Sebe, & M. Welling (Eds.), *Computer vision – ECCV 2016* (pp. 646–661). Springer International Publishing.
5. Mooney, P. (2018). Blood cell images.
6. Tan, M., & Le, Q. V. (2019). Efficientnet: Rethinking model scaling for convolutional neural networks. *CoRR*, abs/1905.11946.
7. Territo, M (2022). Eosinophilic disorders - blood disorders.
8. Territo, M. (2022). Lymphocytic leukocytosis - blood disorders.
9. Territo, M. (2022). Lymphocytopenia - blood disorders.
10. Territo, M. (2022). Monocyte disorders - blood disorders.
11. Territo, M. (2022). Neutropenia - blood disorders.
12. Territo, M. (2022). Neutrophilic leukocytosis - blood disorders.
13. Zoph, B., Vasudevan, V., Shlens, J., & Le, Q. V. (2017). Learning transferable architectures for scalable image recognition. *CoRR*, abs/1707.07012.

Chapter 5
CNN for Skin Cancer Classification

5.1 Introduction to Skin Cancer

The most widespread kind of cancer is skin cancer [9]. Sunbathers and others who work or play sports outside are the ones most likely to get skin cancer. Because they have less melanin than those with darker skin, those with fair skin are highly susceptible to most types of skin cancer. Melanin, a protective pigment found in the epidermis, aids in shielding the skin from ultraviolet (UV) rays. But those with dark skin and those whose skin hasn't received a lot of sun exposure are also susceptible to skin cancer development. Furthermore, skin cancers can appear years after x-ray treatment or exposure to carcinogens (for example, ingestion of arsenic).

Skin cancer typically appears in sun-exposed regions of the body, such as the scalp, face, lips, ears, neck, chest, arms, and hands in women, as well as the legs. But it may also develop on parts of your body that are infrequently exposed to sunlight, such as your palms, the skin just below your finger or toenail, and your genital region.

Every year, there are over 5.4 million new cases of skin cancer being diagnosed in the US [9].

These are the three most common forms of skin cancer:

- Basal cell carcinoma
- Melanoma
- Squamous cell carcinoma

Long-term sun exposure is a contributing factor in the development of these three kinds.

5.1.1 Basal Cell Carcinoma

Basal cell carcinomas make up around 80% of all skin malignancies (also called basal cell cancers) [2]. These malignant tumors typically develop in parts of your body that are exposed to the sun, such your face or neck.

Basal cell cancer may manifest as:

- A lump that is pearly or waxy
- A scar-like lesion that is flat, flesh-colored or brown.
- A sore that bleeds or scabs, which heals but could reappear

5.1.2 Squamous Cell Carcinoma

Squamous cell carcinomas account for around 2 out of 10 skin cancer cases [2]. These cancers begin in the flat cells of the epidermis' upper (outer) layer. Squamous cell carcinoma most usually affects your hands, cheeks, ears, and other sun-exposed regions of your body. People with darker skin are more prone to develop squamous cell carcinoma in places that are rarely exposed to sunlight.

Squamous cell carcinoma could manifest as:

- A red, hard nodule
- A flat lesion with a crusty, scaly exterior

5.1.3 Melanoma

Melanoma can appear anywhere on your body, in normally healthy skin or in a mole that has already been there [2]. Men who are impacted by melanoma typically develop it on their faces or trunks. In women, this particular kind of cancer most frequently manifests itself on the lower legs. Melanoma may also develop on skin that hasn't been exposed to the sun. Everyone is at risk of developing melanoma, regardless of skin color. People with darker skin tend to get melanoma on their palms or soles, or under their fingernails or toenails.

Signs of melanoma include:

- A sizable patch that is brown with darker speckles.
- A mole that bleeds, grows in size, color, or texture.
- A tiny lesion that has an uneven border and areas that can seem pink, white, blue, or blue-black in color.
- An uncomfortable, burning, or itchy lesion
- Dark lesions on your hands, feet, fingertips, or toes, or on the mucous membranes lining your mouth, nose, vagina, or anus

The majority of skin malignancies are treatable, particularly when caught early. In the initial stages, skin cancers do not show any signs. Because of this, it is important to have a doctor look at any strange skin growth that grows or persists for more than a few weeks.

5.2   Skin Cancer Dataset

The dataset contains 2637 dermoscopic training images, 324 validation images and 336 test images of unique benign and malignant skin lesions from various patients [4]. Each image is associated with one of these individuals using a unique patient identifier. All malignant diagnoses have been confirmed via histopathology, and benign diagnoses have been confirmed using either expert agreement, longitudinal follow-up, or histopathology.

The dataset was generated by the International Skin Imaging Collaboration (ISIC) and images are from the following sources: Hospital Clínic de Barcelona, Medical University of Vienna, Memorial Sloan Kettering Cancer Center, Melanoma Institute Australia, University of Queensland, and the University of Athens Medical School [4].

5.3   Classifying Skin Cancer

CNNs has a very wide range of applications in a series of fields such as image recognition, lesion detection and feature analysis [1]. It is intensively used in medical field for lesion classification purposes [5]. The network structure of CNN mainly includes: convolutional layer, down sampling layer and fully connected layer.

The pooling operation is generally conducted after the convolution layer, and its objective is to reduce the amount of data processing while retaining useful information, thus improving the generalization ability of the network [8]. As network continues to deepen, parameters which require updating increase enormously. Some redundant parameters occur and they can be trained on unwanted or incorrect features, leading to common overfitting problems. In addition, a Flatten operation is commonly used in the transition from the convolutional layer to the fully connected layer, which could "flatten" the input, that is, to make the multi-dimensional input become one-dimensional [7]. Therefore, the problem of overfitting became much more severe in CNN.

To prevent overfitting, a global average pooling (GAP) method was proposed in 2014, by Min Lin et al. [6]. GAP is widely used in many classical multi-layer CNN networks, such as ResNet, ShuffleNet, and DenseNet. In a common convolutional neural network, the convolutional layer before the fully connected layer can extract features of the input image. After that, compared to the traditional method which is connecting the full connected layer and then performing activation function, GAP is used to replace the fully connected layer, thus reducing huge parameters to be trained in network [6].

Although GAP mitigates the problem of overfitting well, there are still a series of drawbacks. First, GAP is a global pooling method. Regardless of the width and height of the input layer, it will be numerically averaged, which obviously makes the information of high-level feature maps lose some spatial features. Second, compared with Flatten, GAP is essentially a structural regularization method. It reduces too many parameters and this excessive regularization tends to reduce the model fitting degree and speed.

Instead for skin cancer classification, we will utilize line average pooling (LAP) instead of GAP. LAP uses random column averaging or row averaging method to process feature maps of different channels, thereby realizing two-dimensionality of three-dimensional data. Then, we transform the two-dimensional data into a one-dimensional long vector through the Flatten method. While ensuring the reduction of parameters, LAP retains more spatial features, thereby improving the fitting degree of the model. We will show the difference in performance of the three different pooling methods—flatten, GAP and LAP—on CNNs, and visualize the convergence of the model after 100 epochs [3].

5.3.1 Data Pre-processing

Data processing is a necessary preprocessing at the beginning of experiment. Firstly, when we downloaded these pictures from ISIC archive datasets in benign and malignant categories, these pictures were directly downloaded into two folders named their categories. After that, we use image.open() function from the PIL module to read the pictures and reshaped the size of these pictures to 224×224 by resize function. Then, we use ImageDataGenerator() function to generate train, validation, and test data. In statistic, the distribution of the training set and the proportion of different datasets are as follows (Fig. 5.1).

The function ImageEnhance in PIL and random function in numpy were utilized to change saturation, brightness, contract, and sharpness of these images randomly. As shown in Fig. 5.2, the images after color enhancement were saved to richen our training data, which could avoid over-fitting by providing some noises in training data to increase robustness of training model (Fig. 5.3).

After the preprocessing discussed above, we designed convolutional neural networks (CNNs) by adding the convolution and pooling layers and set relevant parameters. There are some details of the convolution and pooling layers (Fig. 5.4).

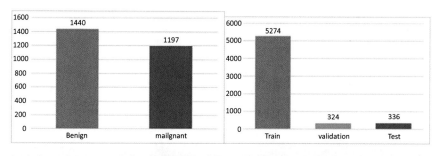

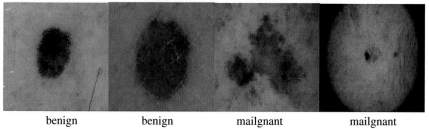

benign   benign   mailgnant   mailgnant

Fig. 5.1 The distribution and the examples of the data set

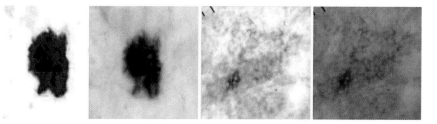

Fig. 5.2 The examples of color enhancement images

5.3.2 Convolution and Pooling Layer

In the first convolutional layer, we used 3×3 filter, and the parameter of padding was set to be "same", so the 224×224 image remained the same shape for the output. Besides, The max pooling layer outputs the maximum value of each 2×2 matrix. The output of this layer is 112×112 images, as in Fig. 5.5.

Totally, there are 6 convolution layers and 6 max pooling layers in our neutral network.

Layer (type)	Output Shape	Param #
conv2d (Conv2D)	(None, 224, 224, 16)	448
batch_normalization (BatchN ormalization)	(None, 224, 224, 16)	64
max_pooling2d (MaxPooling2D)	(None, 112, 112, 16)	0
dropout (Dropout)	(None, 112, 112, 16)	0
conv2d_1 (Conv2D)	(None, 112, 112, 32)	4640
batch_normalization_1 (Batc hNormalization)	(None, 112, 112, 32)	128
max_pooling2d_1 (MaxPooling 2D)	(None, 56, 56, 32)	0
dropout_1 (Dropout)	(None, 56, 56, 32)	0
conv2d_2 (Conv2D)	(None, 56, 56, 64)	18496
batch_normalization_2 (Batc hNormalization)	(None, 56, 56, 64)	256
max_pooling2d_2 (MaxPooling 2D)	(None, 28, 28, 64)	0
dropout_2 (Dropout)	(None, 28, 28, 64)	0
conv2d_3 (Conv2D)	(None, 28, 28, 128)	73856
batch_normalization_3 (Batc hNormalization)	(None, 28, 28, 128)	512
max_pooling2d_3 (MaxPooling 2D)	(None, 14, 14, 128)	0
dropout_3 (Dropout)	(None, 14, 14, 128)	0
conv2d_4 (Conv2D)	(None, 14, 14, 512)	590336
batch_normalization_4 (Batc hNormalization)	(None, 14, 14, 512)	2048
max_pooling2d_4 (MaxPooling 2D)	(None, 7, 7, 512)	0
dropout_4 (Dropout)	(None, 7, 7, 512)	0

Fig. 5.3 The structure of CNN

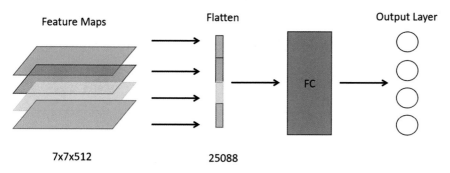

Fig. 5.4 The process of flatten method

flatten (Flatten)	(None, 25088)	0
dense (Dense)	(None, 256)	6422784
dropout_5 (Dropout)	(None, 256)	0
dense_1 (Dense)	(None, 128)	32896
dropout_6 (Dropout)	(None, 128)	0
dense_2 (Dense)	(None, 2)	258

```
=================================================================
Total params: 7,146,722
Trainable params: 7,145,218
Non-trainable params: 1,504
```

Fig. 5.5 Network structure of flatten and fully-connected layers

5.3.3   Final Pooling Operation

Flatten

In one of our three models, we use flatten method as a final pooling layer in order
that convolution layers could be connected well to the fully connected layers. In
Fig. 5.4 below, the convolution layers provide feature maps with size $7 \times 7 \times 512$
(height, width, channel), we use flatten function to flatten the map into 1D vector
which has a length of 25,088. Then we pass these number of neuro points to several
dense layers so that we can produce an output layer with 2 neurons for classification
purpose. The values of prediction are processed by softmax function afterwards.

Global Average Pooling

We adopt GAP method to replace flatten method. When the feature maps are provided with shape $7 \times 7 \times 512$, GAP helps to average all the values on every channel. In other words, each channel of feature map becomes a global averaged value, thus producing a 1D vector with length 512. Then this vector would be fed directly to the output layer instead of being passed through the fully connected layers.

Line Average Pooling

Line Average Pooling (LAP) is the method we proposed, which should serve as an alternative to GAP. It is expected to prevent overfitting problem which occurs severely when applying flatten. It should also be useful in fitting the data with faster speed and avoid underfitting problem which occurs frequently when using GAP. When the feature maps are generated from the early convolution layers with shape $7 \times 7 \times 512$, LAP would average the value in every channel. This is done by averaging the values along horizontal axis or vertical axis randomly. Therefore, we can change the 3D feature maps into 2D feature maps with shape 7×512. After that, these 2D maps are flattened into 1D vector with length 3584. These data points are then fed to the output layer. Softmax is used as well to output prediction values (Figs. 5.6 and 5.7).

Loss Function and Optimizer

After building the network structure, we choose the appropriate loss function and optimizer according to the requirements. Considering that this is a typical binary classification problem, binary cross entropy is chosen as our loss function, which

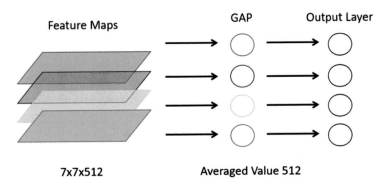

Fig. 5.6 The process of GAP method

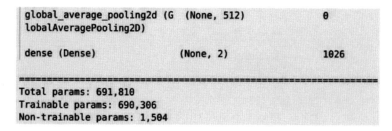

```
global_average_pooling2d (G   (None, 512)                    0
lobalAveragePooling2D)

dense (Dense)                 (None, 2)                   1026

=================================================================
Total params: 691,810
Trainable params: 690,306
Non-trainable params: 1,504
```

Fig. 5.7 Network structure of GAP

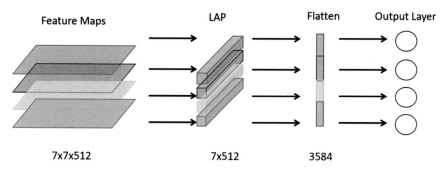

Feature Maps   LAP   Flatten   Output Layer

7x7x512   7x512   3584

Fig. 5.8 The process of LAP method

```
global_line_pooling2d (Glob   (None, 7, 512)                 0
alLinePooling2D)

flatten (Flatten)             (None, 3584)                   0

dense (Dense)                 (None, 2)                   7170

=================================================================
Total params: 697,954
Trainable params: 696,450
Non-trainable params: 1,504
```

Fig. 5.9 Network structure of LAP

can well calculate the error caused by forward propagation. The equation for calculation is as follows:

$$L(w) = -\frac{1}{N}\sum_{i=1}^{N}[y_i log f(x_i) + (1 - y_i) log(1 - f(x_i))]$$

L is value of loss, w is weight of the model, N equals 2 for two labels y1 = 0 and y2 = 1, f(x) is the probability that the output belongs to the y label (Figs. 5.8, 5.9, and 5.10).

$$Iteration : t = t + 1$$
$$m_t = \beta_1 m_{t-1} + (1 - \beta_1) g_t$$
$$V_t = \beta_2 V_{t-1} + (1 - \beta_2) g_t^2$$
$$\alpha_t = \alpha * \sqrt{1 - \beta_2^t / (1 - \beta_1^t)}$$
$$w_{t+1} = w_t - \alpha_t \frac{m_t}{\sqrt{V_t} + \epsilon}$$

Fig. 5.10 The algorithm of Adam optimizer

Table 5.1 Train accuracy (100 epochs) and best test accuracy

	Flatten	LAP	GAP
Train	0.9928	0.9738	0.9423
Test	0.8312	0.8756	0.8811

After that, in order to make the loss reach the global optimum point as much as possible and avoid falling into the local optimum point, we use the Adam optimizer. The Adam optimizer combines the advantages of AdaGrad (for processing sparse gradients) and RMSProp (for processing online data). It is better in adjusting the learning rate of parameters automatically, improving the training speed, as well as improving stability. Its algorithm is as follows:

5.3.4 Training

Training Procedure

To illustrate and compare the performance of LAP against GAP, we trained 3 CNN networks using different final pooling operations: Flatten, LAP and GAP. The epoch was set to 100 so that each model would achieve convergence. As the ISIC Skin Cancer dataset was split into training, validation and testing, we train our models on the training set and record the loss and accuracy on the validation set, thus plotting figures afterwards. Finally, we evaluated our trained models on test set (Table 5.1).

Result

From our accuracy and loss curves, it can be seen that on the training set, the Flatten method has the best model fitting ability and fitting speed, LAP has almost the same ability, while GAP is not effective, and the model features are not widely extracted (Figs. 5.11 and 5.12).

In the analysis on the validation set, the Flatten method cannot effectively prevent overfitting, especially the loss curve oscillates violently at the end. However, the

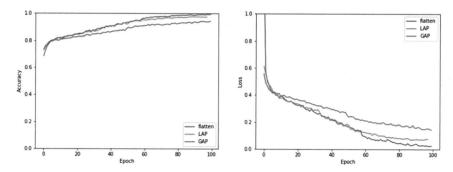

Fig. 5.11 Training: Accuracy curve (left) and loss curve (right)

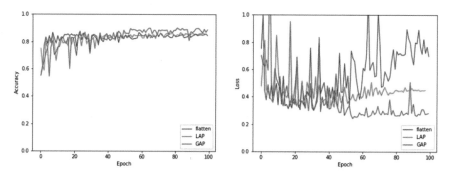

Fig. 5.12 Validation: Accuracy curve (left) and loss curve (right)

GAP method can effectively reduce the overfitting of the model, and achieve the best accuracy and the lowest loss. The LAP algorithm proposed by us is also very effective in preventing overfitting and avoiding the oscillation of the loss curve. The stability and generalization ability of the model are good.

Looking at the accuracy on train set after running 100 times of epoch, model using Flatten reaches 99.28%, LAP reaches 97.38% and GAP reaches 94.23%. Comparing the best accuracy on test set, the model using Flatten reaches 83.12%, LAP reaches 87.56% and GAP reaches 88.11%.

This result is consistent with the analysis of the loss and accuracy curves, that is, GAP is the best in solving the problem of overfitting, LAP also has good generalization ability, and Flatten has serious overfitting problem.

Improvement of the Model

As can be seen from the results, model using LAP witnessed better generalization ability than model using Flatten. However, compared with GAP, LAP still has slightly overfitting problem due to the added parameters. Therefore, we made small changes to LAP model. We manually added L2 normalization to the loss function to speed up weight decaying. In addition, we attempted to find the optimal hyperparameter of dropout rate to mitigate overfitting. The dropout rate was reassigned from 0.2 to 0.3 for the second experiment. Batchnormlazation was utilized just as the first model.

$$J(\theta) = \frac{1}{2m} \left[\sum_{i=1}^{m} (y_i - h_\theta(x_i))^2 + \lambda \sum_{j=1}^{n} \theta_j^2 \right]$$

The result is that on the test set, LAP reaches 88.42% while GAP reaches 88.17%. It shows that after the adoption of additional regularization, LAP can even perform better than GAP with its good generalization ability and convergence speed.

5.3.5   Conclusion

We show that a structural regularizaiton method called Line Average Pooling can help improve performance for skin cancer classification. LAP replaces traditional fully-connected layers and is capable of performing random row or column-wise averaging of feature maps. In order to demonstrate the performance of LAP, we compared the result of using LAP, Flatten and GAP on the Skin cancer dataset for binary classification. The result shows that models using Flatten, LAP and GAP reaches 83.12%, 87.56% and 88.11% on the test set. With additional regularization methods used, LAP even performs better than GAP. When compiling the model, LAP saves a lot of model parameters, so it can greatly mitigate overfitting problem. Comparing against GAP, LAP adopts milder structural regularization. We have shown that LAP is better in learning the features and improving convergence speed for skin cancer classification.

References

1. Akter, M., Hossain, M. S., Ahmed, T. U., & Andersson, K. (2021). Mosquito classification using convolutional neural network with data augmentation. In P. Vasant, I. Zelinka, & G.-W. Weber (Eds.), *Intelligent computing and optimization* (pp. 865–879). Springer International Publishing.
2. American Cancer Society. What are basal and squamous cell skin cancers? Types of skin cancer.
3. Chen, Z., Du, Y., & Teoh, T. T. (2022). Line average pooling: A better way to handle feature maps on cnn for skin cancer classification. In *2022 Asia conference on cloud computing, computer vision and image processing (3CVIP)*.
4. Fanconi, C. (2019). Skin cancer: Malignant vs. benign.
5. Kasinathan, G., Jayakumar, S., Gandomi, A. H., Ramachandran, M., Fong, S. J., & Patan, R. (2019). Automated 3-d lung tumor detection and classification by an active contour model and cnn classifier. *Expert Systems with Applications, 134*(C), 112–119.

6. Lin, M., Chen, Q., & Yan, S. (2013). Network in network, 2013. arxiv:1312.4400. Comment: 10 pages, 4 figures, for iclr2014.
7. Wang, Z. J., Turko, R., Shaikh, O., Park, H., Das, N., Hohman, F., Kahng, M., & Chau, D. H. (2020). Cnn 101: Interactive visual learning for convolutional neural networks. In *Extended abstracts of the 2020 CHI conference on human factors in computing systems*, CHI EA '20 (pp. 1–7). Association for Computing Machinery.
8. Wang, Z. J., Turko, R., Shaikh, O., Park, H., Das, N., Hohman, F., Kahng, M., & Chau, D. P. (2021). Cnn explainer: Learning convolutional neural networks with interactive visualization. *IEEE Transactions on Visualization & Computer Graphics, 27*(02), 1396–1406.
9. Wells, G. L. (2022). Overview of skin cancer - skin disorders.

Chapter 6
CNN for Diabetic Retinopathy Detection

6.1 Introduction to Diabetic Retinopathy

Diabetic retinopathy is an eye disorder that can affect people with diabetes. It develops when there is damage to the blood vessels in the retina brought on by high blood sugar levels. These vessels have the potential to expand and leak. Alternatively, they might shut, preventing blood from flowing. On occasion, though, aberrant new blood vessels may form on the retina. One's vision may get impaired as a result of all of these changes. The most common reason for blindness in people of working age in industrialized countries is diabetic retinopathy. An estimated 93 million individuals would be impacted by this disease.

According to the World Health Organization, there are 422 million cases of diabetes globally [9]. Long-term diabetes is a risk factor for diabetic retinopathy (DR). Nearly 40–45% of Americans with diabetes are in some stage of the illness [1]. If DR is discovered early enough, the progression of visual impairment can be delayed or prevented. However, this can be challenging because the condition usually exhibits few symptoms until it is too late for effective therapy.

In its early stages, diabetic retinopathy shows no symptoms. As diabetic retinopathy worsens, you may experience symptoms like:

- seeing an increase in floaters
- experiencing blurred vision
- having eyesight that shifts from fuzzy to clear at times
- seeing empty or dark regions in your field of vision
- not having good night vision
- observing that colors seem faded or washed out
- becoming blind

Currently, diagnosing DR involves an in-depth manual examination of digital color fundus pictures of the retina by a qualified practitioner. By the time human reviewers have submitted their reviews, which is frequently a day or two later,

T. T. Teoh, *Convolutional Neural Networks for Medical Applications*, SpringerBriefs in Computer Science, https://doi.org/10.1007/978-981-19-8814-1_6

the delayed results have caused lost follow-up, misunderstandings, and postponed treatment [1].

Clinicians are able to diagnose DR if there are lesions present that are related with the vascular anomalies that are induced by the illness. Although this strategy works, it has substantial resource requirements. In regions with high rates of diabetes in the local population and a need for DR detection, the necessary skills and equipment are typically insufficient. The infrastructure needed to stop DR-related blindness will get even more inadequate as the number of people with diabetes rises.

The necessity for a thorough and automated DR screening approach has long been acknowledged, and prior initiatives have made excellent strides utilizing image classification, pattern recognition, and machine learning. The objective of the task is to push an automated detection system to its absolute limit using color fundus photography, ideally producing models with realistic clinical potential.

6.2   Diabetic Retinopathy Dataset

The data of this experiment came from the APTOS2019 dataset of Kaggle Community Competition, which contained 5590 high-resolution retinal images diagnosed by professional ophthalmologists with different degrees of severity [1]. The dataset contains high-resolution retina images taken under a variety of imaging conditions. A left and right field is provided for every subject. Images are labeled with a subject id as well as either left or right (e.g. 1_left.jpeg is the left eye of patient id 1).

The presence of diabetic retinopathy in each image has been rated by a clinician on a scale of 0–4, according to the following scale: 0—No DR (Fig. 6.1a); 1—Mild (Fig. 6.1b); 2—Moderate (Fig. 6.1c); 3—Severe (Fig. 6.1d); 4—Proliferative DR (Fig. 6.1e)

In the medical field, when a convolutional neural network is used for multiple classifications, the number of classification categories and image quality have a great influence on the accuracy of classification. The amount of sample image data of different types in this dataset is seriously unbalanced, with the amount of normal data being more than 10 times that of diseased data, which is shown in the Fig. 6.2

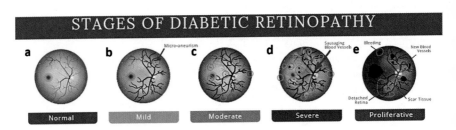

Fig. 6.1 (a) Normal DR (b) mild DR (c) moderate DR (d) severe DR (e) proliferative DR

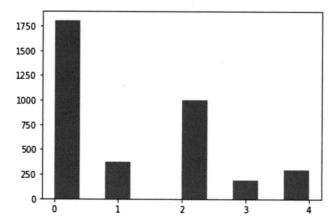

Fig. 6.2 Distribution of five levels of DR samples

Table 6.1 Distribution of classes

Class name	Degree of DR	Numbers
Class 0	Normal	1874
Class 1	Mild	396
Class 2	Moderate	1005
Class 3	Severe	219
Class 4	Proliferative	257

and Table 6.1. In addition, the fundus image will generate noise in the process of collection due to the factor of environment.

6.2.1 Non-proliferative Diabetic Retinopathy

The initial stages of diabetic eye illness is non-proliferative diabetic retinopathy (which ranges from scale 1 to 3 of our dataset). It is common among diabetics.

With NPDR, microscopic blood vessels leak, causing the retina to enlarge. It is referred to as macular edema when the macula becomes swollen. This is the leading cause of blindness in persons with diabetes [2].

Additionally, blood vessels in the retina may collapse with NPDR. We refer to this as macular ischemia [2]. When that occurs, the macula is not able to receive blood. In the retina, small specks known as exudates can occasionally occur. These can also impair your vision.

Your eyesight will be fuzzy if you have NPDR.

6.2.2   Proliferative Diabetic Retinopathy

In our dataset, proliferative diabetic retinopathy (PDR), the more severe stage of diabetic eye disease and is represented by a scale of 4. This occurs as new blood vessels begin to form in the retina. This process is known as neovascularization [2]. These delicate young arteries frequently bleed into the vitreous. If they bleed only a little bit, you could notice a few black floaters in the blood. A lot of bleeding might completely impair eyesight.

Scar tissue may develop from these new blood vessels. Scar tissue can harm the macula or result in a detached retina.

PDR is extremely dangerous and can impair both your central and peripheral (side) vision.

The photos in the dataset were captured using various camera models and configurations, which may have an impact on how left and right look. Some of the photographs depict the retina anatomically (macula on the left, optic nerve on the right for the right eye). Others are displayed in the manner of what a microscope condensing lens would reveal (i.e. inverted, as one sees in a typical live eye exam). Typically, there are two techniques to determine whether a picture is upside down:

If the macula, which is the tiny, black core region, is somewhat higher than the optic nerve's midline, the image is said to be inverted. It is not inverted if the macula is lower than the optic nerve's midline.

The picture is not flipped if it has a notch (square, triangle, or circle) on one of the sides. Without a notch, it is flipped.

There will be noise in the labels and the photos, just as in any real-world data collection. Images might be out of focus, overexposed, underexposed, or contain artifacts. The creation of resilient algorithms that can operate in the midst of noise and fluctuation is one of the main goals of this task.

6.3   Classifying Diabetic Retinopathy

6.3.1   Diabetic Retinopathy

Diabetic retinopathy (DR) is one of the most grievous oculopathies, with potential possible effects of causing blindness [4–8]. The etiopathogenesis of DR is that high glucose toxicity caused by diabetes gives birth to changes in the nervous system and capillaries of the eye [4, 7, 8]. Usually, DR could be divided into two main classifications: Nonproliferative (NPDR) and Proliferative (PDR) [4, 6–8]. According to the degree of the lesion, DR could also be classified into 5°, normal, mild, moderate, severe, and proliferative, respectively from 0 to 4 to represent the degree [4, 6–8]. Without early diagnosis and timely treatment, the initial NPDR or low-level DR might finally develop to be PDR over time, which is server and get people trapped into a riskier situation [4, 6–8]. Early detection could help human beings aware of DR in time and take measures to protect the vision. However, the mild symptoms might increase the difficulty of the early detection and following corresponding treats of the affected patients in usual traditional manual methods for its limitation due to subjectivity and instability [6–8]. In addition, it will be a huge cost both at the aspect of time and money since manual detection requires the trained experts to perform on the base of their experience. Thus, it seems that vision-based methods through computers gradually become more appropriate alternative choices due to their high efficiency, accuracy, and objectivity compared with the conventional one mentioned before [3].

6.3.2 Deep Learning and Image Identification

With the rapid progress of computer science, Deep Learning, as the main part of artificial intelligence, plays a more and more essential role in almost all fields, especially in the area of medical science. Nowadays in a period of Big Data, information explosion requires people to get prepared to deal with the overwhelming diverse data efficiently. In the field of multiform data, image accounts for more than 70%, which means that as one critical field of Deep Learning, the development of image identification and recognition matters and they have permeated virtually every aspect of people's life [8]. The medical detection of certain diseases with relatively regular and similar could be operated by computer rather than doctors to save cost and improve the efficiency as well as accuracy because there exist unstable factors such as inattention even if the doctor is experienced and specialized [7, 8].

6.3.3 Training

Data Preparation

During the process of collection, the fundus image will generate noise due the collection environment, this would eventually lead to a slow convergence speed of the network and thus failure to reach the target.

In order to solve unbalanced number of retinal image samples and image noise, the image is preprocessed before feeding into the network. Data preprocessing is as follows:

1. Due to the influence of the collection environment, fundus images with partially black or completely black will be collected, and these meaningless data will be processed and reduce the efficiency of the training network, so these data will be deleted.
2. Remove the black edge around the retinal image of the fundus.

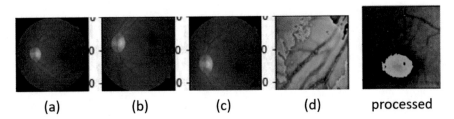

(a)   (b)   (c)   (d)   processed

Fig. 6.3 (a)–(d) The processes of data preparation

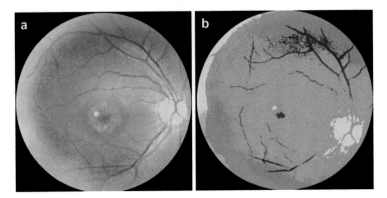

Fig. 6.4 (a) Initial image. (b) After augmentation

3. In order to reduce the computational burden of the simulation experiment, the resolution size of the training data is adjusted to 244 × 244, as shown in Fig. 6.3
4. Due to the imbalance of the amount of data in each category, the data enhancement method is used to increase the number of samples. This is mainly increased by flipping and reviewing images, so that the number of categories in the United States and China is basically the same, so as to solve the problem of sample imbalance, as shown in Fig. 6.3b and c.
5. The image is normalized to reduce the interference caused by uneven light, as shown in Fig. 6.3d.

Additionally, image data preparation has a significant impact on neural network and convolutional neural network model training, as mentioned before, when the sample space or the number of samples is not enough, they will seriously affect the training or lead to the lack of generalization of trained, resulting in relatively low recognition rate and accuracy. Here a method of Data Augmentation to solve this issue is proposed, including changing the brightness and shade, flipping, ZCA whiting (a process to reduce the redundancy of input data), and decentration. The comparison between the initial image and the image after the augmentation is shown in Fig. 6.4a and b.

Setting of the Experiment

The pre-processed data were divided and 66% of the data were used as training set for training network and parameter learning 34% of the data were used as a test set to test the identification and generalization ability of the model.

6.3.4   Result and Evaluation

After an 8-h process of training and testing, the results of this initial image recognition and classification model could be seen and evaluated. The evaluation indicators of the recognition of the classification mainly consist of two parts, accuracy and loss.

Accuracy

The first indicator is the accuracy, which is the ratio of the number of one set of correctly classified image samples to the total expected number of the given set. According to the graphic result, the accuracy on the training set was about 87.89% and the accuracy on the validation set was about 79.72%. From the graphic of both training and validation accuracy, it could be seen that the general overall trend of the accuracy of both kinds was upward even though there existed fluctuation throughout the process (Fig. 6.5).

Loss

Another indicator for evaluation is loss, which is usually used for evaluating the difference between the result distribution and given standard expected distribution and perform quantitative calculation of the extent of this difference. Actually, the cross-entropy function is frequently utilized for such loss function. To be more specific, cross-entropy serves to judge the determine how close the actual output is to the desired output. The cross-entropy of the distribution q relative to a distribution p over a given set is defined as follows:

$$H(p, q) = -E_p[logq]$$

```
Training Loss = 0.512670        Accuracy on Training set = 87.886130% [2902/3302]

Validation Loss = 0.730906      Accuracy on Validation set = 79.722222% [287/360]
```

Fig. 6.5 The accuracy of training set and validation set

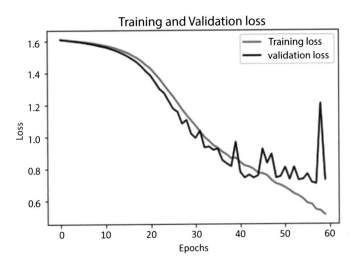

Fig. 6.6 The loss of training set and validation set

where-E_p is the expected value operator with respect to the distribution p. The definition may be formulated using the Kullback–Leibler divergence $D_{KL}(P\|Q)$, divergence of p from q (also known as the relative entropy of p with respect to q).

$$H(p,q) = H(p) + D_{KL}(p\|q)$$

where H(p) is the entropy of p. For discrete probability distributions p and q with the same support χ, this means

$$H(p,q) = -\sum_{x\in\chi} p(x)logq(x)$$

The graph of Fig. 6.6 expresses the two kinds of loss, where the green line represents the training loss and the blue one represents the validation loss. It could be seen that the validation loss remained a slight decrease during about the first 15 epochs and experienced a short but rapid decline during approximately 20–35 epochs. After that, it fluctuated between 0.7 and 1.2 dramatically to the end.

6.3.5   The Optimisation of Convolutional Neural Network

Improvement of the Model

While operations such as convolution, pooling and activation function layers map the original data to the hidden feature space, the fully connected layer serves to

```
#Since we have less data, we will use transfer learning
model = models.resnet34(pretrained = True) #Downloads the model pretrained on Imagenet dataset.

model.fc = nn.Sequential(
    nn.Linear(512,128),
    nn.ReLU(inplace=True),
    nn.Dropout(0.1),
    nn.Linear(128,5),
)
```

Fig. 6.7 Modification of the layer

```
Training Loss = 0.044470      Accurancy on Training set = 98.788613% [326
2/3302]

Validation Loss = 1.738698    Accurancy on Validation set = 83.611111% [30
1/360]
```

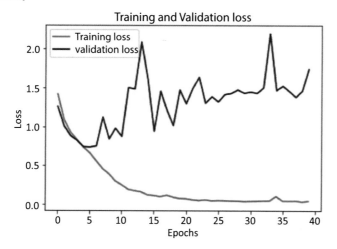

Fig. 6.8 Modified model structure

map the learned "distributed feature representation" to the sample tagging space. To optimize the fit pattern, two new Dropout () functions are added to the fully-connected layer to regularize the overfitting, and the learning rate is adjusted from 0.001 to 0.01 to speed up the fit. Additionally, removing a redundant fully connected layer reduces the computation time required by the model with little impact on accuracy. The modified code is shown in Fig. 6.7.

Results After Improvement

After the operation improvement settings were altered as mentioned before, the results of the improved ResNet34 model could be shown at the aspect of accuracy and loss in Fig. 6.8

As two graphs showed, this improved model could have the over 98% training accuracy and over 83% validation accuracy. However, the loss of the validation was not satisfactory and it was not stable or downward, especially during the latter process, which means that there still existed serious overfitting during the process.

6.3.6   Comparison with Other Models

To objectively evaluate the performance of ResNet34 among CNN, other competitive models, including Densenet121, Alexnet and Inception V3 have also been simulated to obtain the accuracy and loss. Table 6.2 shows the accuracy of each model and Fig. 6.9 show the loss graphic respectively.

Table 6.2 Accuracy of different models

Model name	Accuracy
Densenet121	82.50
Alexnet	71.39
Inception V3	81.11
Resnet34	83.61

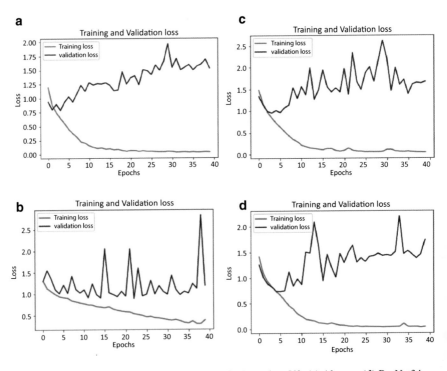

Fig. 6.9 The loss of 4 models. (**a**) Densenet121. (**b**) Inception_V3. (**c**) Alexnet. (**d**) ResNet34

From the results, it could be concluded that ResNet34 is still competitive for its high accuracy.

6.3.7 Conclusion

Diabetes is one of the gradually serious diseases, which might cause other subsequent diseases, including Diabetic Retinopathy. The traditional manual diagnosing is time-consuming and lack of stability compared with advanced automatic visual detection by algorithm. Based on improved Convolutional Neural Network and ResNet34 model, a method of Image Recognition for Diabetic Retinopathy detection is proposed. Results express that the detection accuracy could reach about 83% which is higher than 79% after the optimization. However, the graphic of model loss is unsatisfactory, which means that there exists an overfitting phenomenon during this recognition process [3].

References

1. California Healthcare Foundation and EyePacs. Diabetic retinopathy detection.
2. Gregori, N. Z. (2022). Diabetic retinopathy: Causes, symptoms, treatment.
3. Guo, W., Dong, M., Guo, R., Du, X., Li, X., Zhao, Y., & Teoh, T. T. (2022). Diabetic retinopathy detection method based on improved convolutional neural network using fine-tuning. In *2022 4th international conference on robotics and computer vision (ICRCV)*.
4. Jinfeng, G., Qummar, S., Junming, Z., Ruxian, Y., & Khan, F. G. (2020). Ensemble framework of deep CNNs for diabetic retinopathy detection. *Computational Intelligence and Neuroscience, 2020*, 1–11.
5. Kolla, M., & Venugopal, T. (2021). Efficient classification of diabetic retinopathy using binary cnn. In *2021 International conference on computational intelligence and knowledge economy (ICCIKE)* (pp. 244–247).
6. Li, Q., Peng, C., Ma, Y., Du, S., Guo, B., & Li, Y. (2021). Pixel-level diabetic retinopathy lesion detection using multi-scale convolutional neural network. In *2021 IEEE 3rd global conference on life sciences and technologies (LifeTech)* (pp. 438–440).
7. Qummar, S., Khan, F. G., Shah, S., Khan, A., Shamshirband, S., Rehman, Z. U., Khan, I. A., & Jadoon, W. (2019). A deep learning ensemble approach for diabetic retinopathy detection. *IEEE Access, 7*, 150530–150539.
8. Raj, M. A. H., Mamun, M. A., & Faruk, M. F. (2020). Cnn based diabetic retinopathy status prediction using fundus images. In *2020 IEEE region 10 symposium (TENSYMP)* (pp. 190–193).
9. World Health Organization. Diabetes.

Index

Printed in the United States
by Baker & Taylor Publisher Services